Quick and Effective Workouts

Get Fit Fast with Efficient Exercise Routines

Gary Burke

Quick and Effective Workouts

TABLE OF CONTENTS

Chapter 1: The Science Behind Quick Workouts 6

The Physiology of Short, Intense Exercise 6

Benefits of High-Intensity Interval Training (HIIT) 10

Metabolic Effects of Quick Workouts 14

Comparing Quick Workouts to Traditional Routines 18

Research and Studies Supporting Quick Workouts 23

Chapter 2: Designing Efficient Exercise Routines 28

Principles of Effective Workout Design 28

Balancing Cardio and Strength Training 33

Creating Full-Body Workouts 37

Customizing Workouts for Different Fitness Levels 41

Sample Quick Workout Plans 45

Chapter 3: Quick Cardio Workouts 50

High-Intensity Interval Training (HIIT) 50

Tabata Workouts 54

Plyometrics and Jump Training 58

Circuit Training for Cardio 63

Sample 10- to 20-Minute Cardio Routines 68

Chapter 4: Efficient Strength Training 74

The Basics of Strength Training 74

Compound Movements for Maximum Efficiency 78

Bodyweight Exercises 83

Resistance Band and Dumbbell Workouts 87

Chapter 5: Flexibility and Mobility in Minimal Time 92

The Importance of Flexibility 92

Quick Stretching Routines 96

Dynamic Warm-Ups and Cool-Downs 100

The Physiology of Short, Intense Exercise

Short, intense exercise has risen in popularity due to its efficiency and effectiveness. Understanding the underlying physiology of these workouts reveals why they are so potent and how they can be optimized for maximum benefit. The human body is a complex system, and short, intense exercise leverages several key physiological mechanisms to deliver significant fitness improvements in a fraction of the time of traditional workouts.

At the heart of short, intense exercise is the concept of high-intensity interval training (HIIT). This method alternates between brief periods of maximum effort and lower-intensity recovery periods. The physiology of HIIT revolves around the body's metabolic pathways and energy systems. When you engage in a high-intensity exercise, your body predominantly uses the anaerobic energy system. This system provides quick bursts of energy by breaking down glucose without oxygen, resulting in the production of lactic acid. The accumulation of lactic acid leads to the familiar burning sensation in muscles during intense efforts.

Despite its short duration, HIIT can significantly impact cardiovascular and muscular systems. The rapid, repeated activation of these systems during intense intervals forces the body to adapt in ways that traditional, steady-state exercise does not. One of the primary adaptations is an increase in mitochondrial density. Mitochondria are the powerhouses of cells, responsible for producing energy. More mitochondria mean your muscles can generate energy more efficiently, improving endurance and performance.

Another crucial adaptation involves the cardiovascular system. HIIT has been shown to enhance the heart's stroke volume, which is the amount of blood pumped per heartbeat. This improvement allows the heart to pump more blood with each beat, reducing the overall workload on the heart and increasing cardiovascular efficiency. Additionally, high-intensity exercise improves the elasticity of blood vessels, facilitating better blood flow and reducing blood pressure over time.

The hormonal response to short, intense exercise is another significant factor in its effectiveness. High-intensity efforts stimulate the release of several key hormones, including adrenaline, noradrenaline, and growth hormone. These hormones play vital roles in energy metabolism, fat oxidation, and muscle growth. The surge in adrenaline and noradrenaline increases the breakdown of fat stores, providing a readily available energy source and contributing to fat loss. Growth hormone, on the other hand, promotes muscle repair and growth, enhancing strength and muscle mass.

The metabolic effects of quick workouts extend beyond the exercise session itself. One of the most notable benefits is the post-exercise oxygen consumption, commonly referred to as the afterburn effect. After an intense workout, the body continues to consume oxygen at an elevated rate to restore itself to its pre-exercise state. This process, known as excess post-exercise oxygen consumption (EPOC), increases calorie expenditure for hours after the workout has ended. This extended calorie burn is a significant advantage of short, intense workouts over traditional steady-state exercise.

Comparing quick workouts to traditional routines highlights several advantages. Traditional endurance-based exercises, such as long-distance running or cycling, primarily utilize the aerobic energy system, which relies on a steady supply of oxygen to produce energy. While effective for cardiovascular health and endurance, these workouts often require longer durations to achieve similar benefits to those provided by HIIT. Additionally, the repetitive nature of traditional endurance exercises can lead to overuse injuries and may not provide the same level of muscular and metabolic adaptations as high-intensity training.

Research and studies supporting the efficacy of HIIT and other forms of short, intense exercise are plentiful. Numerous studies have demonstrated that HIIT can improve cardiovascular fitness, increase insulin sensitivity, and reduce body fat more effectively than traditional exercise routines. For example, a study published in the   found that just two weeks of HIIT significantly improved mitochondrial function and insulin sensitivity in sedentary adults. Another study in the   reported that HIIT was more effective at reducing visceral fat, the dangerous fat surrounding internal organs, compared to moderate-intensity continuous training.

The physiological benefits of short, intense exercise are not limited to elite athletes or fitness enthusiasts. These workouts can be tailored to suit individuals of all fitness levels, from beginners to advanced. The key is to adjust the intensity and duration of the intervals to match the individual's current fitness level while progressively increasing the challenge as they become fitter.

Incorporating variety into short, intense workouts can further enhance their effectiveness. Different forms of high-intensity training, such as Tabata, plyometrics, and circuit training, target various aspects of fitness and prevent monotony. Tabata, for instance, involves 20 seconds of all-out effort followed by 10 seconds of rest, repeated for four minutes. This method is highly effective at improving both aerobic and anaerobic capacity. Plyometrics, which involve explosive movements like jumping and bounding, enhance muscular power and coordination. Circuit training combines strength and cardio exercises into a single session, promoting overall fitness and calorie burn.

Safety is paramount when engaging in high-intensity exercise, especially for beginners or those with pre-existing medical conditions. It is essential to start with a thorough warm-up to prepare the muscles and cardiovascular system for the upcoming effort. Dynamic stretches and light aerobic activity can increase blood flow and reduce the risk of injury. Listening to your body and allowing adequate recovery time between intense sessions is also crucial to prevent overtraining and injury.

In conclusion, the physiology of short, intense exercise reveals a multitude of benefits that make it a highly effective and efficient workout method. By leveraging the body's metabolic pathways, enhancing cardiovascular and muscular systems, and stimulating beneficial hormonal responses, high-intensity interval training and other forms of quick workouts provide a powerful tool for improving fitness in a time-efficient manner.

With proper implementation and attention to safety, individuals of all fitness levels can reap the rewards of these potent exercise routines.

Benefits of High-Intensity Interval Training (HIIT)

High-Intensity Interval Training (HIIT) has become a cornerstone of modern fitness due to its remarkable efficiency and effectiveness. This training method, characterized by short bursts of intense exercise followed by brief recovery periods, delivers profound benefits that extend well beyond the realms of traditional exercise routines. Understanding these benefits can help individuals of all fitness levels harness the power of HIIT to achieve their health and fitness goals more quickly and effectively.

One of the most significant benefits of HIIT is its superior efficiency in improving cardiovascular health. Traditional cardiovascular exercises, such as jogging or cycling at a steady pace, are effective but often require long durations to yield noticeable results. HIIT, on the other hand, can achieve similar or even superior cardiovascular benefits in a fraction of the time. The intense intervals push the heart to work harder, improving its efficiency and capacity. Over time, this leads to a lower resting heart rate and improved blood circulation, reducing the risk of heart disease and other cardiovascular conditions.

In addition to cardiovascular health, HIIT is exceptionally effective at enhancing metabolic function. The short, intense bursts of activity during HIIT sessions stimulate both aerobic and anaerobic energy systems. This dual engagement not only burns calories during the workout but also elevates the metabolic rate for hours afterward, a phenomenon known as excess post-exercise oxygen consumption (EPOC). EPOC ensures that your body continues to burn calories at an accelerated rate even after the workout has ended, making HIIT a powerful tool for weight loss and fat reduction.

Muscle building and retention are other notable benefits of HIIT. Unlike traditional steady-state cardio, which can sometimes lead to muscle loss due to prolonged catabolic states, HIIT helps preserve and even build muscle mass. The high-intensity intervals stimulate muscle fibers and promote the release of growth hormone, which is vital for muscle repair and growth. This makes HIIT an excellent choice for those looking to improve muscle tone and strength while simultaneously burning fat.

HIIT's impact on insulin sensitivity and glucose metabolism is another significant advantage. Regular HIIT sessions have been shown to improve insulin sensitivity, allowing the body to use glucose more efficiently and reducing the risk of type 2 diabetes. This is particularly beneficial for individuals with insulin resistance or those at risk of developing diabetes. By improving the body's ability to manage blood sugar levels, HIIT contributes to better overall metabolic health.

The adaptability and versatility of HIIT are also key benefits. HIIT can be tailored to suit various fitness levels and preferences, making it accessible to a wide range of individuals. Whether performed on a treadmill, in a swimming pool, with bodyweight exercises, or using resistance equipment, the principles of HIIT remain the same. This flexibility allows individuals to incorporate HIIT into their fitness routines regardless of their current fitness level or available equipment, ensuring that everyone can benefit from this powerful training method.

Mental health benefits are another compelling reason to incorporate HIIT into your fitness regimen. The intense nature of HIIT workouts triggers the release of endorphins, often referred to as "feel-good" hormones. These endorphins can help reduce stress, anxiety, and depression, promoting a more positive mental state. Additionally, the sense of accomplishment that comes from completing a challenging HIIT session can boost self-esteem and confidence, further enhancing mental well-being.

HIIT also has practical advantages in terms of time management. In today's fast-paced world, finding time for a lengthy workout can be challenging. HIIT addresses this issue by providing an effective workout in as little as 20 minutes. This makes it easier for busy individuals to fit exercise into their schedules, ensuring they can still achieve their fitness goals without sacrificing other important aspects of their lives.

The benefits of HIIT extend beyond physical fitness and into the realm of functional fitness. Functional fitness focuses on exercises that mimic everyday activities and improve overall movement efficiency. HIIT often incorporates compound movements that engage multiple muscle groups simultaneously, enhancing coordination, balance, and overall functional strength. This can translate to improved performance in daily tasks, reducing the risk of injury and enhancing quality of life.

Scientific research consistently supports the benefits of HIIT. Numerous studies have demonstrated its effectiveness in improving various aspects of health and fitness. For example, a study published in the found that just two weeks of HIIT significantly improved cardiovascular fitness and mitochondrial function in sedentary adults. Another study in the reported that HIIT was more effective than traditional cardio at reducing abdominal fat, a key risk factor for metabolic diseases.

HIIT's benefits are not limited to young, healthy individuals. Older adults can also reap significant rewards from incorporating HIIT into their routines. Research has shown that HIIT can improve cardiovascular health, muscle mass, and metabolic function in older populations, contributing to healthier aging and increased longevity. The adaptability of HIIT allows it to be modified to suit the needs and capabilities of older adults, ensuring they can exercise safely and effectively.

Despite its many benefits, it's important to approach HIIT with caution, especially for beginners or those with pre-existing health conditions. Starting with a thorough warm-up is crucial to prepare the body for the intense effort ahead and reduce the risk of injury. Beginners should start with shorter intervals and gradually increase the intensity and duration as their fitness improves. Listening to your body and allowing adequate recovery time between sessions is also essential to avoid overtraining and ensure optimal results.

Incorporating HIIT into your fitness routine can provide a multitude of benefits, from improved cardiovascular health and metabolic function to enhanced muscle strength and mental well-being. The efficiency, adaptability, and versatility of HIIT make it an ideal choice for individuals looking to maximize their fitness results in a time-efficient manner. By understanding and leveraging the unique advantages of HIIT, you can transform your fitness journey and achieve your health goals more effectively than ever before.

Metabolic Effects of Quick Workouts

The allure of quick workouts lies in their promise of efficiency without sacrificing results. Amidst busy schedules and the constant search for balance, these brief, intense sessions offer a powerful solution. Understanding the metabolic effects of quick workouts can help you harness their full potential and make informed decisions about incorporating them into your fitness regimen.

At the core of the metabolic benefits of quick workouts is their ability to enhance the body's energy systems. When you engage in high-intensity exercise, your body taps into both aerobic and anaerobic pathways to meet the immediate energy demands. The anaerobic system, which doesn't rely on oxygen, kicks in first, breaking down stored glucose into ATP (adenosine triphosphate), the primary energy currency of cells. This process, known as glycolysis, produces energy rapidly but also leads to the accumulation of lactic acid, which contributes to the familiar muscle burn during intense efforts.

As the workout progresses, the aerobic system takes over, utilizing oxygen to produce ATP more sustainably. This shift engages the mitochondria, the powerhouses of cells, leading to enhanced mitochondrial biogenesis. This means your body increases the number and efficiency of mitochondria, improving your overall capacity to generate energy. Enhanced mitochondrial function translates to better endurance, reduced fatigue, and improved overall metabolic health.

One of the most significant metabolic effects of quick workouts is the phenomenon known as excess post-exercise oxygen consumption (EPOC), or the afterburn effect. After a high-intensity workout, your body continues to consume oxygen at an elevated rate to restore itself to its pre-exercise state. This process involves replenishing energy stores, repairing muscle tissue, and clearing metabolic byproducts like lactic acid. EPOC can elevate your metabolic rate for hours, sometimes up to 24 hours, post-exercise. This means you're burning more calories even when you're not actively working out, making quick workouts highly effective for weight management and fat loss.

Quick workouts also have a profound impact on hormone regulation, which plays a pivotal role in metabolism. High-intensity exercise stimulates the release of several key hormones, including adrenaline, noradrenaline, and growth hormone. Adrenaline and noradrenaline, commonly known as the fight-or-flight hormones, increase heart rate, blood flow to muscles, and the breakdown of fat stores for energy. This hormonal surge not only boosts performance during the workout but also enhances fat oxidation and energy expenditure afterward.

Growth hormone, another critical player, is released in response to the stress of high-intensity exercise. It promotes muscle repair and growth, increases fat metabolism, and helps regulate blood sugar levels. The combined effect of these hormonal responses is a more efficient and effective metabolism, contributing to improved body composition and overall metabolic health.

Insulin sensitivity is another crucial aspect of metabolism that benefits from quick workouts. Insulin is a hormone that regulates blood sugar levels by facilitating the uptake of glucose into cells. High-intensity exercise improves insulin sensitivity, meaning your cells become more responsive to insulin, allowing for better glucose uptake and utilization. Improved insulin sensitivity reduces the risk of type 2 diabetes and other metabolic disorders, making quick workouts a powerful tool for long-term metabolic health.

The impact of quick workouts on metabolic flexibility is also notable. Metabolic flexibility refers to the body's ability to switch between different fuel sources, such as carbohydrates and fats, based on availability and demand. High-intensity exercise trains the body to become more adept at utilizing both glucose and fat for energy. This adaptability not only enhances performance during varied physical activities but also supports overall metabolic health by preventing the over-reliance on any single energy source.

Incorporating quick workouts into your routine can also lead to favorable changes in body composition. The combination of increased calorie burn, enhanced fat oxidation, and improved muscle mass contributes to a leaner, more toned physique. Muscle tissue is metabolically active, meaning it burns more calories at rest compared to fat tissue. By promoting muscle growth and retention, quick workouts help elevate your basal metabolic rate (BMR), the number of calories your body needs to maintain basic physiological functions at rest.

The versatility of quick workouts makes them accessible and practical for individuals with varying fitness levels and goals. Whether your aim is to lose weight, build muscle, or improve overall health, these workouts can be tailored to meet your needs. For beginners, starting with shorter intervals and gradually increasing intensity and duration ensures a safe and effective progression. For more advanced individuals, incorporating a variety of exercises and modalities, such as bodyweight movements, resistance training, and plyometrics, can keep the workouts challenging and engaging.

Despite their brevity, quick workouts can deliver significant cardiovascular benefits. The high-intensity intervals push your heart and lungs to work harder, improving cardiovascular efficiency and endurance. Over time, this leads to a stronger heart, improved circulation, and lower resting heart rate. These cardiovascular adaptations not only enhance athletic performance but also reduce the risk of heart disease and other cardiovascular conditions.

The mental benefits of quick workouts should not be overlooked. The intense nature of these sessions triggers the release of endorphins, often referred to as the body's natural mood enhancers. This endorphin rush can help reduce stress, anxiety, and depression, promoting a more positive mental state. Additionally, the sense of accomplishment that comes from completing a challenging workout can boost self-esteem and confidence, further enhancing mental well-being.

For those concerned about time constraints, quick workouts offer a practical solution. In a world where time is often the most limited resource, the ability to achieve significant metabolic and fitness benefits in just 20 to 30 minutes is invaluable. This makes it easier to maintain a consistent exercise routine, even with a busy schedule, ensuring long-term adherence and success.

Safety and proper technique are paramount when engaging in high-intensity exercise, especially for beginners. A thorough warm-up is essential to prepare the muscles and cardiovascular system for the demands of the workout. Dynamic stretches and light aerobic activity can increase blood flow and reduce the risk of injury. It's also important to listen to your body and allow adequate recovery time between sessions to prevent overtraining and ensure optimal results.

In conclusion, the metabolic effects of quick workouts are profound and multifaceted. From enhanced energy systems and elevated post-exercise calorie burn to improved hormone regulation and insulin sensitivity, these workouts offer a powerful and efficient way to improve overall metabolic health. Their versatility, accessibility, and practicality make them an ideal choice for individuals seeking to maximize their fitness results in a time-efficient manner. By understanding and leveraging the unique advantages of quick workouts, you can transform your fitness journey and achieve your health goals more effectively than ever before.

Comparing Quick Workouts to Traditional Routines

In the bustling world we live in, finding time for a lengthy workout can often seem like an insurmountable challenge. This is where quick workouts come into play, offering a time-efficient alternative to traditional exercise routines.

Understanding the differences between quick workouts and traditional routines can help you make informed decisions about which approach best suits your lifestyle and fitness goals.

Quick workouts, often referred to as high-intensity interval training (HIIT) or circuit training, are designed to maximize effort in a short amount of time. These sessions typically range from 15 to 30 minutes and consist of brief, intense bursts of exercise followed by short rest periods. This approach contrasts sharply with traditional routines, which usually involve longer, steady-state activities like jogging, cycling, or weightlifting sessions that can last an hour or more.

One of the primary benefits of quick workouts is their efficiency. For busy individuals, the appeal of fitting a complete workout into a short time frame is undeniable. You can achieve significant health and fitness benefits without dedicating large chunks of your day to exercise. This efficiency is not just about saving time; it's also about maximizing the effectiveness of every minute spent working out.

In terms of cardiovascular benefits, quick workouts have been shown to be highly effective. The intense nature of these sessions pushes your heart rate to higher levels, improving cardiovascular fitness in a shorter period. Studies have demonstrated that HIIT can improve cardiovascular health as effectively as traditional endurance training, despite requiring significantly less time. This makes quick workouts an excellent option for those looking to boost heart health without committing to extended exercise sessions.

From a metabolic perspective, quick workouts offer unique advantages. The high-intensity intervals stimulate both aerobic and anaerobic energy systems, leading to improved metabolic flexibility. This means your body becomes better at switching between different fuel sources, enhancing overall energy efficiency. Additionally, the phenomenon of excess post-exercise oxygen consumption (EPOC) ensures that your body continues to burn calories at an elevated rate long after the workout has ended. This afterburn effect is less pronounced in traditional steady-state exercises, making quick workouts more effective for fat loss and weight management.

Quick workouts also have a significant impact on muscle building and retention. The varied and intense nature of these sessions engages multiple muscle groups, promoting muscle growth and strength. Traditional routines often focus on isolated muscle groups, which can be effective but may require longer sessions to achieve comprehensive results. By incorporating compound movements and high-intensity intervals, quick workouts provide a full-body workout that can lead to better muscle tone and overall strength.

Despite their many benefits, quick workouts are not without their challenges. The high intensity can be demanding, particularly for beginners or those with certain health conditions. It's essential to approach these workouts with caution, starting with manageable intervals and gradually increasing intensity as your fitness level improves. Proper warm-up and cool-down routines are also crucial to prevent injury and ensure optimal performance.

Traditional routines, on the other hand, have their own set of advantages. They are often less intimidating for beginners, providing a more gradual introduction to physical activity. Steady-state exercises like walking, jogging, or cycling are accessible and can be adjusted to suit various fitness levels.

These routines also allow for longer periods of sustained activity, which can be beneficial for building endurance and cardiovascular health over time.

For those focused on specific fitness goals, traditional routines can offer more targeted training. Bodybuilders, for instance, may prefer longer weightlifting sessions that isolate specific muscle groups to achieve hypertrophy. Endurance athletes might opt for extended cardio sessions to build stamina and aerobic capacity. The structure of traditional routines provides the flexibility to tailor workouts to individual needs and objectives.

Mental health benefits are another area where traditional routines excel. The repetitive, rhythmic nature of activities like running or cycling can be meditative, helping to reduce stress and improve mental clarity. The longer duration of these sessions also provides an opportunity for reflection and mental relaxation, which can be particularly valuable in our fast-paced world.

However, the time commitment required for traditional routines can be a significant drawback for many people. Finding an hour or more for exercise can be challenging, leading to skipped workouts and inconsistent training. This is where the practicality of quick workouts shines, offering a viable solution for maintaining a regular exercise routine despite a busy schedule.

When comparing quick workouts to traditional routines, it's essential to consider individual preferences and lifestyle factors. For some, the high-energy, fast-paced nature of quick workouts is highly motivating and aligns well with their fitness goals. For others, the steady, predictable rhythm of traditional routines provides a sense of structure and stability that is equally valuable.

Incorporating a combination of both approaches can often yield the best results. For instance, you might choose to do quick workouts during the week when time is limited, and longer traditional sessions on weekends or days off. This hybrid approach allows you to enjoy the benefits of both methods while keeping your routine varied and engaging.

Ultimately, the choice between quick workouts and traditional routines should be guided by your personal fitness goals, preferences, and lifestyle. Both approaches have their merits and can contribute to improved health and fitness. The key is to find a routine that you enjoy and can stick with consistently, as adherence is the most critical factor in achieving long-term success.

In conclusion, quick workouts and traditional routines each offer unique benefits and challenges. Quick workouts provide time-efficient, high-intensity training that can boost cardiovascular health, enhance metabolism, and build muscle in a short period. Traditional routines offer a more gradual, targeted approach that can improve endurance, build specific muscle groups, and support mental health. By understanding the strengths and limitations of each method, you can make informed decisions about your fitness journey and create a balanced, effective exercise regimen that fits your life.

Research and Studies Supporting Quick Workouts

The appeal of quick workouts has surged in recent years, driven by the promise of achieving substantial fitness benefits in a fraction of the time required for traditional exercise routines. This trend isn't just a product of modern marketing; it is firmly grounded in a growing body of scientific research that underscores the efficacy of short, high-intensity exercise sessions. Understanding the research and studies supporting quick workouts can provide valuable insights into their benefits and inform how they might be effectively incorporated into a fitness regimen.

One of the most compelling pieces of evidence supporting quick workouts comes from research on high-intensity interval training (HIIT). HIIT involves alternating short bursts of intense exercise with periods of rest or low-intensity activity. A landmark study published in the found that just three sessions of HIIT per week, each lasting only about 20 minutes, significantly improved participants' cardiovascular endurance, insulin sensitivity, and muscle oxidative capacity. The study demonstrated that these brief sessions could elicit changes typically associated with much longer periods of traditional endurance training.

Further supporting the cardiovascular benefits of quick workouts, a study in the highlighted the efficiency of HIIT in improving heart health. Researchers found that participants who engaged in 10-minute HIIT sessions, three times a week for six weeks, experienced similar improvements in cardiovascular fitness as those who undertook 150 minutes of moderate-intensity steady-state exercise per week. This evidence suggests that quick workouts can be a viable alternative for individuals seeking to enhance heart health without the time commitment of longer exercise sessions.

The metabolic effects of quick workouts have also been extensively studied. One notable research published in examined the impact of a HIIT protocol on metabolic rate and fat oxidation. The study found that participants who performed 20-minute HIIT sessions experienced a significant increase in their resting metabolic rate (RMR) for up to 24 hours post-exercise. This phenomenon, known as excess post-exercise oxygen consumption (EPOC), indicates that quick workouts can boost metabolism and enhance fat burning long after the workout has ended, making them particularly effective for weight management.

Another aspect of metabolism that benefits from quick workouts is insulin sensitivity. Improved insulin sensitivity means that the body can more effectively regulate blood sugar levels, reducing the risk of type 2 diabetes. Research published in demonstrated that just two weeks of HIIT significantly improved insulin sensitivity in young, sedentary adults. This improvement was comparable to that seen with traditional endurance training, highlighting the potential of quick workouts to positively impact metabolic health in a short amount of time.

Muscle strength and endurance are also areas where quick workouts have shown substantial benefits. A study in the

compared the effects of HIIT and traditional

resistance training on muscle strength and hypertrophy. The results indicated that HIIT, which incorporated bodyweight exercises and plyometrics, was as effective as traditional weightlifting in increasing muscle mass and strength over an eight-week period. This finding is particularly relevant for individuals looking to build muscle but who may not have access to a gym or extensive equipment.

The psychological benefits of quick workouts should not be overlooked. Exercise is well-documented to improve mental health, and quick workouts are no exception. A study in found that participants who engaged in 20-minute HIIT sessions reported significant reductions in stress and anxiety levels. The intense nature of HIIT appears to trigger the release of endorphins, the body's natural mood elevators, which can help alleviate symptoms of depression and anxiety.

Additionally, the adaptability of quick workouts makes them accessible for a wide range of fitness levels and lifestyles. Research published in the compared traditional endurance training with a modified HIIT program designed for older adults and individuals with chronic conditions. The study found that the HIIT program, which included lower-intensity intervals and longer rest periods, was both safe and effective in improving cardiovascular health and functional capacity in these populations. This adaptability underscores the versatility of quick workouts and their potential to benefit a broad spectrum of individuals.

Despite the extensive evidence supporting the benefits of quick workouts, it's essential to consider the quality and design of these studies. Most research on HIIT and quick workouts involves controlled environments and specific protocols, which may not perfectly translate to real-world settings. However, the consistency of positive outcomes across various studies provides a robust foundation for the efficacy of quick workouts.

For beginners looking to incorporate quick workouts into their routine, it's crucial to start gradually and focus on proper technique to avoid injury. High-intensity exercises can be demanding, and without adequate preparation, there's a risk of overexertion. A study in the

emphasized the importance of a proper warm-up and cool-down to prepare the body for the demands of high-intensity exercise and aid in recovery afterward. This approach can help mitigate the risk of injury and ensure a safe, effective workout experience.

Moreover, the social aspect of quick workouts can enhance adherence and enjoyment. Group HIIT classes, which have gained popularity in recent years, offer a sense of community and motivation that can be particularly beneficial for those new to exercise. A study in   found that participants in group exercise programs reported higher levels of motivation and enjoyment compared to those who exercised alone, leading to better adherence and long-term commitment to their fitness routines.

Incorporating quick workouts into a comprehensive fitness plan can provide a balanced approach that leverages the benefits of both high-intensity and traditional exercises. For instance, combining HIIT sessions with moderate-intensity activities like walking or cycling can ensure a well-rounded fitness regimen that addresses cardiovascular health, muscle strength, and overall well-being. This hybrid approach can also prevent monotony and keep workouts engaging, reducing the likelihood of burnout.

Ultimately, the growing body of research supporting quick workouts highlights their potential as a time-efficient, effective alternative to traditional exercise routines. By understanding the scientific evidence and practical applications, individuals can make informed decisions about incorporating quick workouts into their fitness journey. Whether the goal is to improve cardiovascular health, enhance metabolic function, build muscle, or boost mental well-being, quick workouts offer a versatile and accessible solution that can fit seamlessly into even the busiest of schedules.

In summary, the extensive research and studies supporting quick workouts provide compelling evidence of their efficacy across various health and fitness domains. From cardiovascular improvements and metabolic enhancements to muscle strength and mental health benefits, quick workouts offer a powerful, efficient alternative to traditional exercise routines. By incorporating these findings into practical, actionable advice, individuals can harness the benefits of quick workouts to achieve their fitness goals and lead healthier, more active lives.

Principles of Effective Workout Design

Designing an effective workout plan can seem like a daunting task, especially for beginners. However, understanding and applying a few core principles can transform this process into a manageable and even enjoyable endeavor. These principles guide the structure, intensity, and progression of your workouts, ensuring you achieve your fitness goals efficiently and safely.

One of the foundational principles of workout design is specificity. This principle emphasizes that the body adapts to the specific type and amount of stress placed on it. For instance, if your goal is to improve cardiovascular endurance, your workout should focus on activities like running, cycling, or swimming, which challenge the heart and lungs. Conversely, if strength building is your objective, resistance training with weights or body-weight exercises should be prioritized. The specificity principle ensures that your workouts are directly aligned with your fitness goals, maximizing the effectiveness of your efforts.

Another crucial principle is progressive overload. This concept involves gradually increasing the intensity, duration, or frequency of your workouts to continually challenge your body. Without progressive overload, your body will adapt to the existing level of stress, leading to a plateau in fitness gains. Progressive overload can be achieved by adding more weight, increasing the number of repetitions, extending the duration of your cardio sessions, or even reducing rest intervals between sets. The key is to make incremental changes that push your boundaries while allowing adequate recovery.

The principle of variation is also important for effective workout design. Incorporating a variety of exercises and training methods not only prevents boredom but also ensures comprehensive development across different muscle groups and fitness components. For example, combining strength training with cardio, flexibility exercises, and balance work can lead to more balanced overall fitness. This variation can also help prevent overuse injuries that might result from repetitive motions and provide mental stimulation, keeping you motivated and engaged.

Recovery is a vital yet often overlooked principle. Effective workout design must include adequate rest and recovery periods to allow your body to repair and strengthen itself between sessions. Overtraining can lead to fatigue, decreased performance, and increased injury risk. Scheduling regular rest days and ensuring quality sleep are essential components of a balanced workout plan. Additionally, incorporating active recovery, such as light stretching or low-intensity activities, can aid in muscle repair and reduce soreness.

Another key principle is individualization. Everyone's body responds differently to exercise based on factors like genetics, fitness level, age, and injury history. Tailoring your workout plan to your unique needs and abilities can optimize results and reduce the risk of injury. For instance, beginners might start with basic movements and lower intensity, gradually progressing as their fitness improves. Consulting with a fitness professional can provide personalized guidance and adjustments to your plan.

The principle of balance ensures that your workout regimen addresses all major muscle groups and fitness components. Neglecting certain areas can lead to muscular imbalances, poor posture, and increased injury risk. A balanced workout plan includes exercises for strength, endurance, flexibility, and mobility. For example, pairing upper body exercises with lower body movements and incorporating both pushing and pulling exercises can promote muscular symmetry. Additionally, integrating core strengthening exercises can enhance stability and overall functional fitness.

Monitoring and adjusting your workouts based on feedback and progress is another critical principle. Regularly assessing your performance and making necessary modifications ensures continuous improvement and helps you stay on track with your goals. This might involve tracking metrics such as weight lifted, distance run, or even subjective measures like energy levels and mood. Adjustments can be made based on this feedback, whether it means increasing intensity, changing exercises, or allowing more recovery time.

Consistency is the bedrock of any effective workout plan. Sporadic or infrequent exercise will not yield significant results. Establishing a regular exercise routine and sticking to it is essential for long-term progress. Consistency builds habits, and over time, these habits can lead to substantial improvements in fitness. Setting realistic and achievable goals, along with a structured schedule, can enhance adherence and make regular exercise a part of your lifestyle.

Goal setting is a powerful tool in workout design. Clear, specific, and measurable goals provide direction and motivation. Whether your aim is to lose weight, build muscle, improve cardiovascular health, or enhance athletic performance, having defined objectives helps structure your workouts and track progress. Goals should be challenging yet attainable, and it's helpful to break them down into short-term and long-term targets. Celebrating small victories along the way can also boost motivation and commitment.

Mind-body connection plays a significant role in effective workout design. Paying attention to your body's signals during exercise can prevent injury and optimize performance. This involves being mindful of form and technique, recognizing signs of fatigue, and adjusting intensity as needed. Developing a strong mind-body connection enhances the quality of your workouts and ensures that you're working efficiently and safely towards your goals.

Incorporating functional movements into your workout plan is another principle that can enhance overall fitness. Functional exercises mimic everyday activities and improve strength, balance, and coordination in a practical context. Movements like squats, lunges, and push-ups engage multiple muscle groups and joints, promoting better movement patterns and reducing injury risk in daily life. Functional training not only boosts physical fitness but also enhances your ability to perform routine tasks with ease and efficiency.

The principle of enjoyment should not be underestimated. Finding joy in your workouts increases the likelihood of long-term adherence. Engaging in activities that you find fun and fulfilling can transform exercise from a chore into a rewarding experience. Whether it's dancing, hiking, playing a sport, or attending group fitness classes, choosing activities you love helps maintain motivation and consistency. The more you enjoy your workouts, the more likely you are to stick with them and reap the benefits.

Nutrition and hydration are essential components of a well-rounded workout plan. Proper fueling before and after exercise can enhance performance, recovery, and overall results. Consuming a balanced diet rich in whole foods provides the necessary nutrients for energy, muscle repair, and growth. Staying hydrated is equally important, as dehydration can impair performance and recovery. Developing a nutrition plan that complements your workout regimen ensures that your body has the resources it needs to perform at its best.

Finally, patience and realistic expectations are crucial for effective workout design. Fitness improvements take time, and it's important to set realistic timelines for achieving your goals. Recognizing that progress may be gradual and that setbacks are a natural part of the journey can help maintain motivation and prevent frustration. Celebrating small milestones and focusing on the positive changes, however incremental, reinforces the commitment to your fitness plan.

By understanding and applying these principles, you can design an effective and sustainable workout plan tailored to your individual needs and goals. Specificity, progressive overload, variation, recovery, individualization, balance, monitoring, consistency, goal setting, mind-body connection, functional movements, enjoyment, nutrition, hydration, and patience all play crucial roles in crafting a successful fitness journey. These principles provide a comprehensive framework that ensures your workouts are both effective and enjoyable, setting the stage for long-term health and fitness.

Balancing Cardio and Strength Training

Balancing cardio and strength training is essential for creating a well-rounded fitness program that enhances overall health, improves performance, and reduces the risk of injury. Striking the right balance between these two types of exercise can be challenging, but with a clear understanding of their benefits and how they complement each other, you can develop an effective and sustainable workout routine.

Cardio, short for cardiovascular exercise, is any activity that raises your heart rate and increases blood circulation throughout the body. Running, cycling, swimming, and dancing are all popular forms of cardio. This type of exercise is known for its benefits in improving heart health, boosting endurance, burning calories, and aiding in weight management. Regular cardio workouts help strengthen the heart and lungs, making daily activities easier and reducing the risk of chronic diseases such as heart disease, stroke, and diabetes.

Strength training, on the other hand, focuses on building muscle mass, strength, and endurance. It involves exercises that use resistance, such as weightlifting, body-weight exercises, and resistance band workouts. Strength training is crucial for maintaining muscle mass, increasing metabolic rate, improving bone density, and enhancing overall functional fitness. It helps you perform daily tasks more efficiently and reduces the risk of injuries by strengthening muscles, tendons, and ligaments.

To create a balanced workout routine, it's important to integrate both cardio and strength training in a way that aligns with your fitness goals and lifestyle. Here are some practical strategies to help you achieve this balance:

First, assess your fitness goals. Whether you're aiming to lose weight, build muscle, improve endurance, or enhance overall health, your goals will determine the emphasis you place on cardio versus strength training. For example, if weight loss is your primary objective, you might prioritize cardio workouts to burn calories while incorporating strength training to build muscle and boost metabolism. Conversely, if you're looking to build muscle, strength training will take precedence, with cardio serving as a complement to ensure cardiovascular health and endurance.

Scheduling your workouts is another critical aspect of balancing cardio and strength training. A well-structured workout plan typically includes both types of exercise spread throughout the week. For beginners, a common approach is to alternate between cardio and strength training days. For instance, you might perform cardio on Monday, Wednesday, and Friday, and strength training on Tuesday, Thursday, and Saturday. This allows for adequate recovery between sessions and ensures that you're not overworking any particular muscle group.

Combining cardio and strength training in a single session is also a viable option, especially for those with limited time. Circuit training, which involves alternating between cardio and strength exercises with minimal rest, is an effective way to achieve this. For example, you might perform a series of strength exercises like squats, push-ups, and rows, interspersed with short bursts of cardio such as jumping jacks or high knees.

This approach provides a comprehensive workout that targets multiple fitness components simultaneously.

Intensity and duration are key factors to consider when balancing cardio and strength training. High-intensity interval training (HIIT) is a popular method that combines short, intense bursts of cardio with strength exercises. HIIT workouts are efficient and can be completed in a relatively short amount of time while delivering significant benefits for both cardiovascular fitness and muscle strength. Alternatively, you might opt for longer, steady-state cardio sessions on some days and dedicate other days to focused strength training.

Listening to your body is essential in any workout routine. Pay attention to how your body responds to different types of exercise and adjust accordingly. If you feel excessively fatigued or sore, it may be a sign that you need more rest or that you're overtraining a particular aspect of your fitness. Balancing cardio and strength training also involves adequate recovery time, which is crucial for muscle repair and growth. Incorporating rest days and ensuring proper nutrition and hydration will support your overall fitness progress.

Variety is another important element in balancing cardio and strength training. Mixing up your workouts not only prevents boredom but also ensures that you're challenging your body in different ways. For cardio, try incorporating various activities like running, cycling, swimming, or group fitness classes. For strength training, use a mix of free weights, machines, resistance bands, and body-weight exercises. Variety keeps your workouts interesting and helps prevent plateaus by continuously challenging your muscles and cardiovascular system.

Monitoring your progress is a valuable practice in maintaining a balanced workout routine. Keep track of your workouts, noting the types of exercises, duration, intensity, and how you feel before and after each session. This information can help you identify patterns, make adjustments, and ensure that you're progressing towards your fitness goals. Regularly reviewing and updating your workout plan based on your progress and feedback allows for continual improvement and adaptation.

It's also important to remember that balance doesn't mean equal time spent on cardio and strength training. The ratio will vary based on your individual goals, fitness level, and preferences. Some people might find that a 60-40 split in favor of strength training works best for them, while others might prefer a more even distribution. The key is to find a balance that works for you and supports your overall fitness objectives.

Incorporating flexibility and mobility exercises into your routine can further enhance the balance between cardio and strength training. Stretching, yoga, and foam rolling are excellent ways to improve flexibility, reduce muscle tension, and prevent injuries. These activities complement both cardio and strength workouts by promoting better movement patterns and aiding in recovery.

Lastly, maintaining a positive mindset and staying motivated is crucial for long-term success. Setting realistic and achievable goals, celebrating small milestones, and finding enjoyment in your workouts can help you stay committed. Remember that fitness is a journey, and finding a balance that works for you is an ongoing process. Be patient with yourself and open to making adjustments as needed.

By integrating both cardio and strength training into your workout routine, you can achieve a balanced and comprehensive fitness program that supports your overall health and well-being. Each type of exercise offers unique benefits, and together, they create a synergistic effect that enhances your physical capabilities and quality of life. Whether you're a beginner or an experienced exerciser, finding the right balance between cardio and strength training will help you reach your fitness goals and enjoy a healthier, more active lifestyle.

Creating Full-Body Workouts

Balancing cardio and strength training is essential for creating a well-rounded fitness program that enhances overall health, improves performance, and reduces the risk of injury. Striking the right balance between these two types of exercise can be challenging, but with a clear understanding of their benefits and how they complement each other, you can develop an effective and sustainable workout routine.

Cardio, short for cardiovascular exercise, is any activity that raises your heart rate and increases blood circulation throughout the body. Running, cycling, swimming, and dancing are all popular forms of cardio. This type of exercise is known for its benefits in improving heart health, boosting endurance, burning calories, and aiding in weight management. Regular cardio workouts help strengthen the heart and lungs, making daily activities easier and reducing the risk of chronic diseases such as heart disease, stroke, and diabetes.

Strength training, on the other hand, focuses on building muscle mass, strength, and endurance. It involves exercises that use resistance, such as weightlifting, body-weight exercises, and resistance band workouts. Strength training is crucial for maintaining muscle mass, increasing metabolic rate, improving bone density, and enhancing overall functional fitness. It helps you perform daily tasks more efficiently and reduces the risk of injuries by strengthening muscles, tendons, and ligaments.

To create a balanced workout routine, it's important to integrate both cardio and strength training in a way that aligns with your fitness goals and lifestyle. Here are some practical strategies to help you achieve this balance:

First, assess your fitness goals. Whether you're aiming to lose weight, build muscle, improve endurance, or enhance overall health, your goals will determine the emphasis you place on cardio versus strength training. For example, if weight loss is your primary objective, you might prioritize cardio workouts to burn calories while incorporating strength training to build muscle and boost metabolism. Conversely, if you're looking to build muscle, strength training will take precedence, with cardio serving as a complement to ensure cardiovascular health and endurance.

Scheduling your workouts is another critical aspect of balancing cardio and strength training. A well-structured workout plan typically includes both types of exercise spread throughout the week. For beginners, a common approach is to alternate between cardio and strength training days. For instance, you might perform cardio on Monday, Wednesday, and Friday, and strength training on Tuesday, Thursday, and Saturday. This allows for adequate recovery between sessions and ensures that you're not overworking any particular muscle group.

Combining cardio and strength training in a single session is also a viable option, especially for those with limited time. Circuit training, which involves alternating between cardio and strength exercises with minimal rest, is an effective way to achieve this. For example, you might perform a series of strength exercises like squats, push-ups, and rows, interspersed with short bursts of cardio such as jumping jacks or high knees. This approach provides a comprehensive workout that targets multiple fitness components simultaneously.

Intensity and duration are key factors to consider when balancing cardio and strength training. High-intensity interval training (HIIT) is a popular method that combines short, intense bursts of cardio with strength exercises. HIIT workouts are efficient and can be completed in a relatively short amount of time while delivering significant benefits for both cardiovascular fitness and muscle strength. Alternatively, you might opt for longer, steady-state cardio sessions on some days and dedicate other days to focused strength training.

Listening to your body is essential in any workout routine. Pay attention to how your body responds to different types of exercise and adjust accordingly. If you feel excessively fatigued or sore, it may be a sign that you need more rest or that you're overtraining a particular aspect of your fitness. Balancing cardio and strength training also involves adequate recovery time, which is crucial for muscle repair and growth. Incorporating rest days and ensuring proper nutrition and hydration will support your overall fitness progress.

Variety is another important element in balancing cardio and strength training. Mixing up your workouts not only prevents boredom but also ensures that you're challenging your body in different ways. For cardio, try incorporating various activities like running, cycling, swimming, or group fitness classes. For strength training, use a mix of free weights, machines, resistance bands, and body-weight exercises. Variety keeps your workouts interesting and helps prevent plateaus by continuously challenging your muscles and cardiovascular system.

Monitoring your progress is a valuable practice in maintaining a balanced workout routine. Keep track of your workouts, noting the types of exercises, duration, intensity, and how you feel before and after each session. This information can help you identify patterns, make adjustments, and ensure that you're progressing towards your fitness goals. Regularly reviewing and updating your workout plan based on your progress and feedback allows for continual improvement and adaptation.

It's also important to remember that balance doesn't mean equal time spent on cardio and strength training. The ratio will vary based on your individual goals, fitness level, and preferences. Some people might find that a 60-40 split in favor of strength training works best for them, while others might prefer a more even distribution. The key is to find a balance that works for you and supports your overall fitness objectives.

Incorporating flexibility and mobility exercises into your routine can further enhance the balance between cardio and strength training. Stretching, yoga, and foam rolling are excellent ways to improve flexibility, reduce muscle tension, and prevent injuries. These activities complement both cardio and strength workouts by promoting better movement patterns and aiding in recovery.

Lastly, maintaining a positive mindset and staying motivated is crucial for long-term success. Setting realistic and achievable goals, celebrating small milestones, and finding enjoyment in your workouts can help you stay committed. Remember that fitness is a journey, and finding a balance that works for you is an ongoing process. Be patient with yourself and open to making adjustments as needed.

By integrating both cardio and strength training into your workout routine, you can achieve a balanced and comprehensive fitness program that supports your overall health and well-being. Each type of exercise offers unique benefits, and together, they create a synergistic effect that enhances your physical capabilities and quality of life. Whether you're a beginner or an experienced exerciser, finding the right balance between cardio and strength training will help you reach your fitness goals and enjoy a healthier, more active lifestyle.

Customizing Workouts for Different Fitness Levels

Customizing workouts for different fitness levels is crucial for ensuring that exercise routines are effective, safe, and engaging. Whether you're a beginner just starting your fitness journey, an intermediate looking to build on existing progress, or an advanced athlete aiming to push boundaries, tailoring your workouts to your specific fitness level can make all the difference in achieving your goals.

For beginners, the primary focus should be on building a solid foundation. This involves familiarizing oneself with basic exercises, understanding proper form, and gradually increasing intensity to avoid injury. Starting with body-weight exercises is an excellent approach. Simple movements such as squats, push-ups, and lunges help develop strength, balance, and coordination without the need for equipment. Additionally, incorporating low-impact cardio activities like walking, cycling, or swimming can improve cardiovascular health without overwhelming the body.

When designing a beginner's workout plan, it's important to emphasize consistency over intensity. Aim for shorter sessions, around 20-30 minutes, and gradually increase the duration as fitness improves. A typical week might include three days of strength training, focusing on different muscle groups each session, and two to three days of cardio. Rest days are equally important to allow the body to recover and adapt.

Tracking progress is a motivational tool for beginners. Keeping a workout journal or using a fitness app can help record achievements and identify areas for improvement. Celebrate small milestones, such as completing a set without stopping or running an extra minute, to stay motivated and build confidence.

For those at an intermediate fitness level, the focus shifts towards building on the established foundation and introducing more variety into workouts. Intermediate exercisers are typically comfortable with basic movements and can handle increased intensity and complexity. This is the stage where incorporating resistance training with weights or resistance bands becomes beneficial. Exercises such as deadlifts, bench presses, and rows can be added to the routine to target different muscle groups more effectively.

Variety is key for intermediate fitness enthusiasts to prevent plateaus and maintain interest. Introducing circuit training, where different exercises are performed in sequence with minimal rest, can boost cardiovascular fitness while continuing to build strength. High-intensity interval training (HIIT) is another effective method. HIIT alternates between periods of intense effort and recovery, maximizing calorie burn and improving cardiovascular endurance in a shorter time frame.

Intermediate workouts should also start to include more targeted core exercises. Planks, Russian twists, and leg raises help strengthen the core, which is essential for overall stability and performance in other exercises. Flexibility training, such as yoga or dynamic stretching, is important to maintain joint health and enhance recovery.

Advanced fitness enthusiasts have typically built a high level of strength, endurance, and muscle memory, allowing them to perform complex and high-intensity workouts. At this stage, specificity and goal-oriented training become crucial. Advanced athletes often have specific goals, such as preparing for a competition, achieving a personal record, or mastering a particular skill.

Periodization, or varying the workout intensity and volume over different phases, is essential for advanced training. This approach prevents overtraining and promotes continuous improvement. For example, an advanced strength training program might include cycles of hypertrophy (muscle growth), strength, and power phases, each lasting several weeks.

Advanced workouts often incorporate compound lifts such as squats, deadlifts, and Olympic lifts, which require significant strength and coordination. Plyometric exercises like box jumps and medicine ball throws can enhance explosive power. Additionally, incorporating sport-specific drills or advanced techniques like supersets and drop sets can provide the necessary challenge and variety.

Recovery becomes even more critical at the advanced level. Advanced athletes must pay close attention to their bodies, incorporating rest days, proper nutrition, and recovery techniques such as foam rolling, massage, and adequate sleep to support their intense training regimens.

For all fitness levels, it's important to prioritize safety and listen to your body. Proper warm-up and cool-down routines help prevent injuries and aid in recovery. Hydration and nutrition play vital roles in supporting workout performance and overall health. Staying hydrated and fueling the body with balanced meals rich in protein, carbohydrates, and healthy fats is essential for energy and muscle repair.

Customizing workouts also involves considering individual preferences and lifestyle factors. Some people may thrive on solo workouts, while others find motivation in group classes or working with a personal trainer. Time constraints, access to equipment, and personal interests should all be taken into account when designing a fitness plan. The best workout is one that you enjoy and can consistently commit to.

Adapting workouts to different fitness levels also means being open to progression and regression. As fitness improves, exercises should be modified to maintain challenge and promote growth. Conversely, if an exercise feels too difficult or causes discomfort, it's important to adjust or regress to a more manageable variation. This adaptability ensures that workouts remain effective and enjoyable at every stage of the fitness journey.

Incorporating regular assessments can help track progress and adjust workouts as needed. Fitness assessments might include measuring strength through one-rep max tests, tracking endurance with timed runs or cycles, and evaluating flexibility with mobility tests. These assessments provide valuable feedback and help set realistic, achievable goals.

Community and support can also play significant roles in customizing workouts. Joining a fitness community, whether in-person or online, can provide motivation, accountability, and a sense of belonging. Sharing experiences, challenges, and successes with others can enhance the overall fitness journey and provide valuable insights and encouragement.

Ultimately, customizing workouts for different fitness levels is about creating a personalized, dynamic approach that evolves with your progress. By understanding your current fitness level, setting clear goals, and designing a balanced, varied workout plan, you can achieve sustainable results and maintain a lifelong commitment to health and fitness. Whether you're just starting out or looking to take your training to the next level, a thoughtful, individualized approach will help you reach your full potential and enjoy the many benefits of an active lifestyle.

Sample Quick Workout Plans

Finding the time to exercise can be challenging, but quick workout plans can help you stay on track with your fitness goals even on the busiest days. Whether you have just a few minutes or half an hour, you can still get a meaningful workout that boosts your energy, improves your mood, and contributes to your overall fitness.

One effective approach to quick workouts is High-Intensity Interval Training (HIIT). HIIT involves short bursts of intense activity followed by brief periods of rest or lower-intensity exercise. This method is highly efficient, allowing you to get a full-body workout in a fraction of the time of traditional exercise routines. For example, a simple 20-minute HIIT workout might include exercises like jumping jacks, burpees, mountain climbers, and high knees. You could perform each exercise for 30 seconds, followed by 15 seconds of rest, repeating the circuit several times. This not only burns calories but also improves cardiovascular health and builds muscle.

For those who prefer strength training, a quick 15-minute body-weight workout can be incredibly effective. Focus on compound exercises that work multiple muscle groups simultaneously. A sample plan could include squats, push-ups, plank holds, and lunges. Performing three sets of each exercise with minimal rest in between can provide a solid strength workout. For instance, you might do 15 squats, 10 push-ups, a 30-second plank hold, and 10 lunges on each leg, then repeat the circuit three times. This approach ensures you engage major muscle groups, promoting muscle growth and endurance.

If you're looking for a balanced routine that combines both cardio and strength, a 30-minute workout can fit the bill. Start with a 5-minute warm-up, such as brisk walking or light jogging, to prepare your body for exercise and reduce the risk of injury. Follow this with 20 minutes of alternating between cardio and strength exercises. For example, you could do 2 minutes of jumping rope or running in place, followed by 1 minute of a strength exercise like squats or push-ups. Repeat this cycle until you hit the 20-minute mark, then cool down for 5 minutes with stretching exercises to improve flexibility and aid recovery.

Flexibility and mobility are often overlooked but are essential components of a well-rounded fitness routine. A quick 10-minute yoga or stretching session can be integrated into your day to enhance flexibility, reduce muscle tension, and improve overall movement quality. Simple yoga poses like downward dog, child's pose, and cat-cow stretches can be done in a short time frame and provide significant benefits. Alternatively, a series of dynamic stretches, such as leg swings, arm circles, and hip openers, can prepare your body for physical activity or help you unwind after a long day.

For those who spend a lot of time at a desk, incorporating short movement breaks throughout the day can counteract the negative effects of prolonged sitting. Set a timer to remind yourself to stand up every hour and perform a quick 2-minute routine. This could include a combination of standing stretches, light cardio such as marching in place, and strength exercises like desk push-ups or chair squats. These mini-workouts can boost circulation, enhance focus, and contribute to your daily physical activity goals.

Another efficient way to get a workout in is by using minimal equipment that you can keep at home or in the office. Resistance bands are versatile and portable, making them perfect for quick strength-training sessions. A 20-minute resistance band workout might include exercises like banded squats, rows, chest presses, and bicep curls. You can perform each exercise for 12-15 reps, moving quickly from one to the next to keep your heart rate up and maximize the workout's effectiveness.

Incorporating quick workouts into your routine doesn't always require structured exercise sessions. Everyday activities can also count towards your fitness goals. For instance, take the stairs instead of the elevator, walk or bike to work if possible, or engage in active hobbies like gardening or playing with your kids. These activities add up over time and contribute to your overall fitness.

When designing quick workout plans, it's essential to listen to your body and adjust the intensity based on your fitness level and how you're feeling that day. If you're new to exercise or returning after a break, start with shorter, less intense sessions and gradually build up as your fitness improves. Conversely, if you're more advanced, you can increase the intensity by adding weights, increasing the duration of high-intensity intervals, or shortening rest periods.

Consistency is key when it comes to fitness. Even short workouts, when done regularly, can lead to significant improvements in strength, endurance, and overall health. Aim to incorporate quick workouts into your daily routine, whether it's first thing in the morning to kickstart your day, during a lunch break for a midday energy boost, or in the evening to wind down and relieve stress.

Motivation can be a challenge, especially when time is limited. Setting specific, achievable goals can help keep you on track. For example, aim to complete a certain number of quick workouts each week or set a goal to improve your performance in a particular exercise. Tracking your progress, whether through a fitness app, journal, or simple calendar, can also provide a sense of accomplishment and encourage you to stay consistent.

Involving others can make quick workouts more enjoyable and hold you accountable. Find a workout buddy, join a fitness class, or participate in online challenges. Sharing your fitness journey with others can provide support, encouragement, and a sense of community, making it easier to stick with your routine.

Quick workouts are an excellent way to stay active and maintain your fitness goals, even with a busy schedule. By incorporating a variety of exercises and keeping the intensity high, you can maximize the benefits of your workout in a short amount of time. Remember to listen to your body, adjust as needed, and stay consistent. With a little creativity and commitment, you can fit effective workouts into any day, no matter how hectic it may be.

High-Intensity Interval Training (HIIT)

High-Intensity Interval Training (HIIT) has rapidly gained popularity due to its efficiency and effectiveness in improving fitness, burning calories, and enhancing cardiovascular health. This training method alternates between short bursts of intense activity and periods of lower-intensity exercise or rest. The appeal of HIIT lies in its ability to deliver a comprehensive workout in a relatively short amount of time, making it ideal for those with busy schedules.

Understanding the basics of HIIT is essential before diving into specific routines. A typical HIIT session might last anywhere from 10 to 30 minutes, significantly shorter than traditional workout sessions. The key to HIIT's effectiveness is the intensity. During the high-intensity intervals, you push yourself to near maximum effort, engaging both aerobic and anaerobic systems. This not only maximizes calorie burn during the workout but also elevates your metabolic rate for hours afterward, a phenomenon known as the afterburn effect or excess post-exercise oxygen consumption (EPOC).

The versatility of HIIT is one of its greatest strengths. It can be adapted to various fitness levels and can incorporate a wide range of exercises, from running and cycling to body-weight exercises like burpees and squats. For beginners, starting with a simple format can help ease into the routine. A basic HIIT workout might involve 20 seconds of high-intensity exercise followed by 40 seconds of rest or low-intensity activity. As fitness improves, the work-to-rest ratio can be adjusted to increase the challenge.

Creating a HIIT workout plan tailored to your needs involves selecting exercises that target different muscle groups and alternating them throughout the session. For example, a well-rounded 20-minute HIIT workout could include exercises like jumping jacks, high knees, mountain climbers, and push-ups. Perform each exercise at maximum effort for 30 seconds, followed by 30 seconds of rest. Repeat the circuit until the 20 minutes are up, ensuring you maintain proper form to prevent injury.

Warm-up and cool-down are crucial components of a HIIT workout. Begin with a 5-minute warm-up to prepare your muscles and joints for the intense activity ahead. Dynamic stretches such as leg swings, arm circles, and light jogging are effective warm-up exercises. After completing the HIIT session, spend another 5 minutes cooling down with static stretches like hamstring stretches, quad stretches, and shoulder stretches. This helps reduce muscle soreness and improve flexibility.

One of the significant benefits of HIIT is its ability to improve cardiovascular health. Studies have shown that HIIT can increase VO2 max, which is the maximum amount of oxygen your body can utilize during exercise. This improvement in cardiovascular efficiency means your heart and lungs become stronger and more efficient over time. Additionally, HIIT has been linked to reductions in blood pressure and improvements in cholesterol levels, contributing to overall heart health.

HIIT is also highly effective for weight loss and fat reduction. The intense bursts of activity elevate your heart rate and increase calorie expenditure both during and after the workout. Research indicates that HIIT can help reduce visceral fat, the harmful fat stored around internal organs, which is associated with various health risks. Combining HIIT with a balanced diet can accelerate weight loss and improve body composition.

Incorporating HIIT into your fitness routine doesn't require fancy equipment or a gym membership. Many HIIT workouts can be performed using just your body weight, making it accessible and convenient. However, if you prefer variety or have access to equipment, adding tools like dumbbells, kettlebells, or resistance bands can enhance your workouts. For instance, incorporating kettlebell swings or dumbbell thrusters into your HIIT routine can increase the intensity and target different muscle groups.

Recovery is an essential aspect of HIIT training. Due to the high intensity, your muscles and cardiovascular system need time to recover and adapt. It's recommended to perform HIIT workouts 2-3 times per week, allowing at least 48 hours of rest between sessions. On non-HIIT days, consider incorporating low-intensity activities like walking, yoga, or stretching to stay active and promote recovery.

Listening to your body is crucial when engaging in HIIT. The intensity of the workouts can be demanding, and it's essential to recognize the difference between pushing yourself and overexertion. Signs of overtraining include persistent fatigue, decreased performance, and increased susceptibility to injuries. If you experience any of these symptoms, it's important to take a step back, allow for adequate recovery, and possibly consult with a fitness professional to adjust your training plan.

Variety is key to maintaining motivation and preventing plateaus in your fitness journey. Change up your HIIT workouts regularly by incorporating new exercises, adjusting the work-to-rest ratio, or increasing the duration of the high-intensity intervals. This keeps the workouts challenging and engaging, ensuring continuous progress. For example, if you've been doing a lot of body-weight HIIT, try incorporating a HIIT session on a stationary bike or treadmill to mix things up.

Combining HIIT with other forms of exercise can create a well-rounded fitness program. Strength training, for example, complements HIIT by building muscle, which in turn can improve performance during high-intensity intervals and increase overall calorie burn. Flexibility training, such as yoga or Pilates, can enhance recovery and prevent injuries by improving joint mobility and muscle elasticity.

Nutrition plays a vital role in supporting your HIIT workouts and overall fitness goals. Ensure you're fueling your body with a balanced diet rich in lean proteins, complex carbohydrates, healthy fats, and plenty of fruits and vegetables. Proper hydration is also essential, especially when performing high-intensity activities that cause significant sweating. Drinking water before, during, and after your workouts helps maintain performance and aids in recovery.

Tracking your progress can provide motivation and help you stay on track with your fitness goals. Use a fitness app, journal, or simple notebook to record your workouts, noting the exercises performed, duration, and how you felt. Tracking can help you identify patterns, set new goals, and celebrate your achievements, no matter how small they may seem.

HIIT can also be a fun and social activity. Invite friends or family to join your workouts, or participate in group classes either in person or online. The camaraderie and encouragement from others can make the workouts more enjoyable and provide additional motivation to push through the challenging intervals.

High-Intensity Interval Training is a powerful tool for improving fitness, burning fat, and enhancing overall health. Its efficiency makes it an excellent choice for those with busy schedules, while its adaptability ensures it can be tailored to suit various fitness levels and preferences. By incorporating HIIT into your routine, listening to your body, and maintaining a balanced approach to exercise, nutrition, and recovery, you can achieve remarkable results and enjoy the many benefits of this dynamic training method.

Tabata Workouts

Tabata workouts, named after Japanese scientist Dr. Izumi Tabata, represent a specific form of High-Intensity Interval Training (HIIT) structured to maximize both aerobic and anaerobic benefits in a compact timeframe. Dr. Tabata's research demonstrated that short bursts of intense activity followed by brief rest periods could significantly improve athletic performance and cardiovascular health. This discovery has made Tabata workouts popular among fitness enthusiasts looking for effective, time-efficient training methods.

The core structure of a Tabata workout is deceptively simple: 20 seconds of maximal effort followed by 10 seconds of rest, repeated for 8 rounds, totaling four minutes per exercise.

Despite its brevity, this format is incredibly challenging because it demands peak performance during the work intervals, pushing your body to its limits.

For beginners, selecting the right exercises for a Tabata routine is crucial. Start with basic movements that you are comfortable with and can perform safely at high intensity. Common choices include bodyweight exercises like squats, push-ups, burpees, and mountain climbers. These exercises engage large muscle groups, elevate the heart rate quickly, and can be easily modified to match your fitness level.

To illustrate, a beginner-friendly Tabata workout might consist of four different exercises: jumping jacks, push-ups, squats, and mountain climbers. Perform each exercise for 20 seconds at maximum effort, followed by 10 seconds of rest. After completing all four exercises, repeat the circuit once more to complete the Tabata sequence. This approach ensures a full-body workout while keeping the routine dynamic and engaging.

Warm-up is essential before diving into the intensity of a Tabata workout. Spend 5-10 minutes on light cardio, such as jogging or brisk walking, combined with dynamic stretches like arm circles and leg swings. This preparation increases blood flow to your muscles, enhances flexibility, and reduces the risk of injury.

As you progress, you can incorporate more complex and challenging exercises into your Tabata routine. For example, advanced variations might include kettlebell swings, plyometric movements like jump squats, or compound exercises such as thrusters. These movements not only increase the intensity but also add variety, preventing workout monotony and promoting continuous improvement.

Recovery is a critical component of Tabata training. Due to the high intensity, your muscles and cardiovascular system require adequate time to recuperate. Incorporate rest days between Tabata sessions or alternate with lower-intensity workouts to allow your body to repair and strengthen. Listen to your body and adjust the frequency based on how you feel; overtraining can lead to fatigue and diminished performance.

Nutrition plays a supportive role in maximizing the benefits of Tabata workouts. Fueling your body with a balanced diet rich in proteins, healthy fats, and carbohydrates provides the necessary energy for high-intensity exercises and aids in muscle recovery. Hydration is equally important, especially during intense workouts that cause significant sweating. Drink plenty of water before, during, and after your sessions to maintain optimal performance and prevent dehydration.

Tracking your progress can be highly motivating and help you stay on course with your fitness goals. Keep a workout journal or use a fitness app to record your exercises, the number of rounds completed, and any personal notes about your performance. Regularly reviewing your progress allows you to set new goals, celebrate achievements, and make informed adjustments to your training plan.

Variety is essential in a Tabata workout regimen. Changing exercises regularly not only keeps the workouts exciting but also ensures that different muscle groups are targeted, promoting balanced muscle development and preventing plateaus. For instance, you might alternate between bodyweight exercises, resistance training, and cardio-focused movements in your Tabata sessions.

Tabata workouts can be performed anywhere, making them highly convenient. Whether at home, in a park, or at the gym, all you need is a timer and a small space. This flexibility makes it easier to incorporate regular exercise into a busy schedule, eliminating common barriers to maintaining a consistent fitness routine.

To illustrate the effectiveness of Tabata workouts, consider the story of Mark, a busy professional who struggled to find time for exercise. With a demanding job and family commitments, long workouts were impractical. Discovering Tabata training was a game-changer for him. By dedicating just 20 minutes a few times a week, Mark experienced significant improvements in his cardiovascular fitness, strength, and overall energy levels. The structured, intense nature of Tabata allowed him to make the most of his limited time, achieving results that traditional workouts hadn't provided.

Safety is paramount in any high-intensity workout. Proper form is crucial to avoid injuries, especially when performing exercises at maximum effort. If you're new to a particular movement, take the time to master the technique before incorporating it into your Tabata routine. Consider working with a fitness professional who can provide guidance and ensure you're performing exercises correctly.

Incorporating technology can enhance your Tabata experience. Numerous apps and online platforms offer Tabata timers, guided workouts, and tracking tools that can streamline your training sessions. These resources can provide structure, motivation, and accountability, helping you stay committed to your fitness journey.

Community and social support can also play a significant role in maintaining motivation. Joining a group fitness class or finding a workout buddy can make Tabata sessions more enjoyable and provide a sense of camaraderie. Sharing your progress, challenges, and successes with others can foster a supportive environment that encourages consistency and perseverance.

Tabata workouts, with their high intensity and time efficiency, are an excellent addition to any fitness regimen. By starting with basic exercises, gradually incorporating more challenging movements, and ensuring proper recovery, you can harness the full benefits of this training method. Remember to prioritize safety, maintain a balanced diet, and stay hydrated to support your body through the demands of high-intensity exercise. Embrace the flexibility and variety that Tabata workouts offer, and track your progress to stay motivated and on track with your fitness goals. With dedication and consistency, Tabata training can lead to significant improvements in your overall health and fitness, fitting seamlessly into even the busiest of lifestyles.

Plyometrics and Jump Training

Plyometrics and jump training are dynamic and powerful methods designed to enhance explosive strength, agility, and overall athletic performance. Originating from the Greek word "plyo," meaning "to increase," and "metrics," meaning "to measure," plyometrics focuses on rapid stretching and contracting of muscles to generate maximum force in the shortest time possible. This form of training is particularly beneficial for athletes in sports that require quick bursts of speed and power, such as basketball, volleyball, and track and field.

The underlying principle of plyometrics is the stretch-shortening cycle (SSC), a natural muscle function where a muscle is rapidly stretched (eccentric phase) and then immediately shortened (concentric phase). This cycle enables muscles to generate more force than during a standard contraction, enhancing power output.

A fundamental aspect of plyometric training is jump training, which includes a variety of exercises aimed at improving vertical and horizontal jump performance. These exercises range from basic movements like squat jumps and box jumps to more complex drills such as depth jumps and bounding. Each exercise focuses on different muscle groups and movement patterns, providing a comprehensive workout for developing lower body power.

For beginners, starting with basic plyometric exercises is essential to build a solid foundation and prevent injury. Simple movements such as squat jumps and tuck jumps are excellent starting points. In a squat jump, you lower your body into a squat position and then explosively jump upwards, reaching as high as possible before landing softly and immediately going into the next squat. Tuck jumps involve jumping straight up and bringing your knees towards your chest while in the air, then landing softly and repeating.

Proper technique is crucial in plyometric training to maximize benefits and minimize the risk of injury. When performing any jump exercise, focus on landing softly with your knees slightly bent to absorb the impact. This reduces stress on the joints and promotes better control. Additionally, maintaining a strong core and proper posture throughout the movements ensures stability and efficiency.

As you progress, incorporating more advanced plyometric exercises can further enhance your explosive power. Box jumps, for example, involve jumping onto a sturdy platform or box, which requires greater power and coordination. Depth jumps, another advanced exercise, involve stepping off a box and immediately jumping upon landing, utilizing the stretch-shortening cycle to its fullest extent.

Plyometric training isn't limited to lower body exercises. Upper body plyometrics, such as clap push-ups or medicine ball throws, can significantly enhance upper body power and coordination. In a clap push-up, you perform a standard push-up but push off the ground with enough force to clap your hands before landing softly back in the starting position. Medicine ball throws involve explosively throwing a medicine ball against a wall or to a partner, focusing on generating power from your core and upper body.

A well-rounded plyometric workout should include a variety of exercises targeting different muscle groups and movement patterns. A sample routine might include squat jumps, box jumps, depth jumps, and medicine ball throws. Begin with a thorough warm-up, including dynamic stretches and light cardio to prepare your muscles and joints for the high-impact nature of plyometrics.

Rest and recovery are vital components of any plyometric training program. Due to the intense nature of these exercises, your muscles and nervous system require adequate time to recover and adapt. Incorporate rest days between plyometric sessions and ensure you're getting enough sleep and proper nutrition to support muscle repair and growth. Overtraining can lead to fatigue, decreased performance, and increased risk of injury.

Nutrition plays a significant role in supporting your plyometric training. A balanced diet rich in protein, healthy fats, and carbohydrates provides the energy and nutrients necessary for muscle recovery and performance. Hydration is equally important, as intense workouts can lead to significant fluid loss through sweat. Drinking plenty of water before, during, and after your sessions helps maintain optimal performance and prevents dehydration.

Tracking your progress is an effective way to stay motivated and monitor improvements in your plyometric training. Keep a journal or use a fitness app to record the exercises performed, the number of repetitions, and any personal notes about your performance. Regularly reviewing your progress allows you to set new goals, celebrate achievements, and make informed adjustments to your training plan.

Safety is paramount in plyometric training. Proper form and technique are essential to avoid injuries, especially when performing high-impact exercises. If you're new to plyometrics, consider working with a fitness professional who can provide guidance and ensure you're performing exercises correctly. Additionally, always use appropriate footwear and a safe training environment, such as a gym with cushioned floors or a designated training area.

Incorporating variety into your plyometric workouts helps prevent plateaus and keeps the training engaging. Alternate between different exercises, sets, and repetitions to continually challenge your muscles and improve overall performance. For instance, you might combine lower body plyometrics with upper body exercises in a single session or vary the height and distance of jumps to target different muscle fibers.

Plyometric training is not just for athletes; it can benefit anyone looking to improve their overall fitness and functional strength. By enhancing your explosive power, agility, and coordination, plyometrics can improve your performance in daily activities and other forms of exercise. Whether you're an athlete aiming to gain a competitive edge or an individual seeking to boost your physical fitness, incorporating plyometrics into your routine can yield significant benefits.

To illustrate the transformative power of plyometric training, consider the story of Sarah, a recreational runner who wanted to improve her race times. Incorporating plyometrics into her training regimen, Sarah began with basic exercises like squat jumps and gradually progressed to more advanced drills. Over time, she noticed a marked improvement in her running speed and endurance, as well as a reduction in her risk of injury. The increased power and agility gained from plyometric training translated into better overall performance and confidence in her athletic abilities.

In conclusion, plyometrics and jump training offer a powerful and effective way to enhance explosive strength, agility, and overall athletic performance. By starting with basic exercises, progressing to more advanced movements, and ensuring proper recovery, you can harness the full benefits of this dynamic training method. Prioritize safety, maintain a balanced diet, and stay hydrated to support your body through the demands of high-intensity exercise. Embrace the variety and flexibility of plyometrics, track your progress, and enjoy the journey towards improved fitness and performance. With dedication and consistency, plyometric training can lead to significant improvements in your physical capabilities, fitting seamlessly into your overall fitness regimen.

Circuit Training for Cardio

Circuit training for cardio is a highly effective and engaging way to improve cardiovascular fitness, build strength, and burn calories. This training method involves performing a series of exercises in a sequence, with minimal rest between each exercise. The combination of aerobic and anaerobic activities keeps the heart rate elevated, providing both cardiovascular and muscular endurance benefits.

The versatility of circuit training makes it accessible to individuals of all fitness levels. For beginners, starting with a well-rounded selection of exercises that target different muscle groups is crucial. A balanced circuit might include bodyweight exercises, cardio moves, and light resistance training to ensure a comprehensive workout.

A typical circuit training session might begin with a warm-up to prepare the body for the intense activity ahead. Dynamic stretches and light aerobic exercises such as jogging or jumping jacks can help to increase blood flow to the muscles and improve flexibility. Warming up also reduces the risk of injury by loosening the joints and increasing muscle elasticity.

Once warmed up, the circuit can commence. An effective circuit might include exercises such as push-ups, squats, burpees, lunges, jumping jacks, mountain climbers, and planks. Each exercise is performed for a set duration, typically 30 to 60 seconds, before moving on to the next with minimal rest. This format keeps the heart rate elevated, enhancing cardiovascular endurance while also building strength and stamina.

For example, consider a circuit that includes the following exercises:

Jumping jacks

Push-ups

Bodyweight squats

Mountain climbers

Plank

High knees

Lunges

Burpees

Perform each exercise for 45 seconds, followed by 15 seconds of rest before moving on to the next exercise. After completing all eight exercises, rest for one to two minutes before repeating the circuit two to three more times, depending on your fitness level.

One of the key advantages of circuit training is its efficiency. The combination of cardio and strength exercises allows for a high-intensity workout in a short amount of time. This makes it ideal for individuals with busy schedules who may find it challenging to fit longer workouts into their day. A well-structured 20- to

30-minute circuit training session can provide significant cardiovascular and muscular benefits.

Another benefit of circuit training is its adaptability. Exercises can be easily modified to increase or decrease intensity based on individual fitness levels. For beginners, performing push-ups on the knees or using a chair for support during squats can make the exercises more manageable. As strength and endurance improve, these modifications can be adjusted to increase the challenge.

Incorporating equipment such as dumbbells, resistance bands, or medicine balls can also add variety and increase the intensity of the workout. For example, holding a dumbbell while performing lunges or using a medicine ball for Russian twists can enhance muscle engagement and provide a greater challenge.

Proper form is crucial in circuit training to maximize benefits and prevent injuries. Focus on performing each exercise with control and precision. For instance, when doing squats, ensure that your knees do not extend past your toes, and keep your back straight. During push-ups, maintain a straight line from your head to your heels and engage your core to protect your lower back.

Listening to your body and knowing your limits is essential, especially for beginners. It's better to perform fewer repetitions with proper form than to rush through exercises with poor technique. As your fitness level increases, you can gradually increase the duration and intensity of the exercises.

Recovery is an important aspect of any fitness regimen, and circuit training is no exception. The high-intensity nature of the workout places significant stress on the muscles and cardiovascular system. Incorporating rest days into your routine allows your body to recover and adapt, reducing the risk of overtraining and injury. Additionally, focusing on adequate sleep, hydration, and nutrition supports muscle recovery and overall performance.

Nutrition plays a vital role in supporting circuit training for cardio. Consuming a balanced diet rich in protein, carbohydrates, and healthy fats provides the energy needed for intense workouts and aids in muscle repair and growth. Hydration is equally important, as staying properly hydrated helps maintain performance and prevents fatigue.

Tracking progress can be highly motivating and help you stay on course with your fitness goals. Keeping a workout journal or using a fitness app to record the exercises performed, the duration of each exercise, and any personal notes about your performance can provide valuable insights. Regularly reviewing your progress allows you to set new goals, celebrate achievements, and make informed adjustments to your training plan.

The mental benefits of circuit training should not be overlooked. The fast-paced, varied nature of the workout keeps the mind engaged and can help alleviate stress. The sense of accomplishment from completing a challenging circuit can boost confidence and provide a mental lift, making it an excellent choice for overall well-being.

Consider the story of John, a busy professional who struggled to find time for exercise. With a demanding job and family commitments, long workouts were impractical. Discovering circuit training was a game-changer for him. By dedicating just

20 minutes a few times a week to a well-structured circuit, John experienced significant improvements in his cardiovascular fitness, strength, and energy levels. The efficient, high-intensity nature of circuit training allowed him to make the most of his limited time, achieving results that traditional workouts hadn't provided.

Incorporating variety into your circuit training routine helps prevent plateaus and keeps the workouts exciting. Alternate between different exercises, sets, and repetitions to continually challenge your muscles and improve overall fitness. For instance, you might combine bodyweight exercises with resistance training or add new cardio moves to keep the circuit fresh and engaging.

Circuit training can be performed anywhere, making it highly convenient. Whether at home, in a park, or at the gym, all you need is a small space and minimal equipment. This flexibility makes it easier to incorporate regular exercise into a busy schedule, eliminating common barriers to maintaining a consistent fitness routine.

Community and social support can also play a significant role in maintaining motivation. Joining a group fitness class or finding a workout buddy can make circuit training more enjoyable and provide a sense of camaraderie. Sharing your progress, challenges, and successes with others can foster a supportive environment that encourages consistency and perseverance.

In conclusion, circuit training for cardio offers a highly effective and efficient way to improve cardiovascular fitness, build strength, and burn calories. By starting with a well-rounded selection of exercises, focusing on proper form, and gradually increasing intensity, beginners can safely and effectively incorporate circuit training into their fitness routine. Prioritize safety, maintain a balanced diet, and stay hydrated to support your body through the demands of high-intensity exercise. Embrace the variety and flexibility of circuit training, track your progress, and enjoy the journey towards improved fitness and performance. With dedication and consistency, circuit training can lead to significant improvements in your physical capabilities and overall well-being, fitting seamlessly into even the busiest of lifestyles.

Sample 10- to 20-Minute Cardio Routines

Finding time for exercise can be challenging, but even short cardio routines can significantly impact your overall fitness. Efficient, high-intensity workouts can elevate your heart rate, burn calories, and improve cardiovascular health in as little as 10 to 20 minutes. This chapter outlines several practical and effective routines you can perform anywhere, regardless of your fitness level.

Begin with a warm-up to prepare your body for the workout ahead. Dynamic stretches such as leg swings, arm circles, and light jogging ensure your muscles are ready for action and reduce the risk of injury. A good warm-up should last about three to five minutes.

The first sample routine is a high-intensity interval training (HIIT) workout, perfect for those short on time but looking for maximum results. HIIT alternates between short bursts of intense activity and brief periods of rest or lower-intensity exercise. This method keeps your heart rate up and can burn more calories than steady-state cardio.

Start with a 10-minute HIIT session:

Jumping Jacks (30 seconds): Begin by standing upright with your feet together and your arms at your sides. Jump your feet out to the sides while raising your arms overhead. Quickly return to the starting position and repeat.

Rest (15 seconds): Allow yourself a brief recovery period.

High Knees (30 seconds): Run in place, bringing your knees up to your chest as high as possible. Pump your arms to maintain momentum.

Rest (15 seconds): Catch your breath and prepare for the next exercise.

Burpees (30 seconds): Start standing, then drop into a squat position, placing your hands on the floor. Jump your feet back into a plank position, perform a push-up, and quickly return to the squat position. Finish by jumping explosively into the air.

Rest (15 seconds): Use this time to recover.

Mountain Climbers (30 seconds): Begin in a plank position. Bring one knee towards your chest, then quickly switch legs, as if you are running horizontally.

Rest (15 seconds): Take a moment to breathe.

Squat Jumps (30 seconds): Stand with your feet shoulder-width apart. Perform a squat, and as you rise, jump explosively into the air, landing softly back into the squat position.

Repeat the entire circuit once more for a total of 10 minutes. This routine effectively boosts your cardiovascular fitness and engages multiple muscle groups.

For those with a bit more time, a 20-minute cardio routine can provide an even more comprehensive workout. This routine combines bodyweight exercises and cardio moves, ensuring a balanced and effective session.

Try this 20-minute full-body cardio workout:

Warm-up (3 minutes): Perform dynamic stretches and light jogging to get your blood flowing.

Jump Rope (1 minute): If you have a jump rope, use it to jump continuously. If not, mimic the motion by jumping in place and rotating your wrists.

Rest (30 seconds): Recover and catch your breath.

Push-ups (1 minute): Assume a plank position with your hands slightly wider than shoulder-width apart. Lower your body until your chest nearly touches the floor, then push back up. Modify by performing push-ups on your knees if necessary.

Rest (30 seconds): Take a brief break.

Jump Squats (1 minute): Stand with your feet shoulder-width apart. Perform a squat, then jump explosively into the air. Land softly and immediately go into the next squat.

Rest (30 seconds): Allow yourself some recovery time.

Bicycle Crunches (1 minute): Lie on your back with your hands behind your head and your knees bent. Lift your shoulders off the ground and bring your right elbow towards your left knee while extending your right leg. Switch sides and continue alternating.

Rest (30 seconds): Breathe deeply and prepare for the next exercise.

Lunges (1 minute): Stand with your feet together. Step forward with one leg and lower your body until both knees are bent at a 90-degree angle. Push back to the starting position and switch legs.

Rest (30 seconds): Recover briefly.

Plank (1 minute): Hold a plank position with your body in a straight line from your head to your heels. Engage your core and avoid letting your hips sag.

Rest (30 seconds): Take a moment to rest.

Butt Kicks (1 minute): Run in place, kicking your heels towards your buttocks. Use your arms to maintain momentum.

Rest (30 seconds): Catch your breath.

Tricep Dips (1 minute): Find a sturdy chair or bench. Sit on the edge with your hands gripping the front of the seat. Slide your hips off the edge and lower your body by bending your elbows. Push back up to the starting position.

Rest (30 seconds): Rest briefly.

Side Plank (30 seconds each side): Lie on your side with your elbow directly under your shoulder. Lift your hips to form a straight line from your head to your feet. Hold, then switch sides.

Cool-down (3 minutes): Perform static stretches, focusing on the muscles worked during the routine. Hold each stretch for 20 to 30 seconds to promote flexibility and recovery.

This 20-minute routine is designed to maximize efficiency, targeting all major muscle groups while keeping your heart rate elevated.

For days when you need a quick but effective workout, consider a Tabata-style routine. Tabata training consists of eight rounds of 20 seconds of work followed by 10 seconds of rest, totaling four minutes per exercise. This method can be intense but incredibly effective for improving cardiovascular fitness and muscular endurance.

Try this 10-minute Tabata workout:

Warm-up (2 minutes): Prepare your body with dynamic stretches and light jogging.

Tabata Round 1 (4 minutes): Perform 20 seconds of high knees followed by 10 seconds of rest. Repeat for eight rounds.

Rest (1 minute): Recover and prepare for the next exercise.

Tabata Round 2 (4 minutes): Perform 20 seconds of burpees followed by 10 seconds of rest. Repeat for eight rounds.

Cool-down (2 minutes): Finish with static stretches to aid recovery.

This Tabata routine is highly efficient, pushing your limits in a short amount of time and providing substantial cardiovascular benefits.

Consistency is key to seeing results from these routines. Aim to incorporate these workouts into your weekly schedule, gradually increasing intensity as your fitness improves. Whether you have 10 minutes or 20, these cardio routines are designed to fit into your busy life, ensuring you stay active and healthy.

Listening to your body is crucial. If any exercise causes discomfort or pain, modify the movement or choose a different exercise. Proper form and technique are essential to prevent injuries and maximize the effectiveness of your workout.

Remember, the goal is to challenge yourself while enjoying the process. Short, intense cardio routines can be just as effective as longer workouts, making it easier to stay committed and achieve your fitness goals. By incorporating these routines into your daily life, you can improve your cardiovascular health, boost your energy levels, and maintain a healthy lifestyle.

The Basics of Strength Training

Strength training is a foundational component of fitness that not only builds muscle but also enhances overall health and well-being. It involves the use of resistance to induce muscular contraction, which in turn builds the strength, anaerobic endurance, and size of skeletal muscles. Whether you are lifting weights, using resistance bands, or performing bodyweight exercises, the principles of strength training remain consistent.

The cornerstone of effective strength training is understanding the concept of progressive overload. This principle states that in order to build muscle, you must continuously increase the demands placed on the muscles. This can be achieved by increasing the weight, adding more repetitions, or decreasing the rest time between sets. The body adapts to the stress placed upon it, so progressively challenging the muscles ensures continual improvement.

Form and technique are paramount in strength training. Proper form not only maximizes the effectiveness of the exercise but also minimizes the risk of injury. Each movement should be performed with control, ensuring that the target muscles are engaged throughout the exercise. For example, when performing a squat, the feet should be shoulder-width apart, the back straight, and the knees should not extend past the toes. Engaging the core and maintaining a neutral spine are critical for preventing strain on the lower back.

Warm-up routines are an essential part of any strength training session. A proper warm-up increases blood flow to the muscles, raises body temperature, and prepares the joints for the stress of lifting. Dynamic stretches, such as leg swings and arm circles, are effective for loosening up the muscles and increasing range of motion. Starting with lighter weights or performing bodyweight movements like lunges and push-ups can also serve as a good warm-up.

Compound movements are the backbone of strength training. These exercises, which involve multiple joints and muscle groups, are highly efficient and effective. Key compound movements include squats, deadlifts, bench presses, and pull-ups. These exercises not only build strength but also improve coordination and balance. For instance, the deadlift engages the glutes, hamstrings, lower back, and core, making it one of the most comprehensive strength-building exercises.

Isolation exercises, which target a single muscle group, are also important in a well-rounded strength training program. These exercises, such as bicep curls and tricep extensions, allow for focused development of specific muscles. They are particularly useful for addressing muscle imbalances and enhancing muscle definition. Incorporating a mix of compound and isolation exercises ensures balanced muscle development and prevents overuse injuries.

Rest and recovery play a critical role in strength training. Muscles do not grow during the workout itself but rather during the recovery period. It is essential to allow adequate time for the muscles to repair and grow stronger between training sessions. This typically means resting each muscle group for at least 48 hours before working it again. Adequate sleep, hydration, and nutrition are also key components of the recovery process. Consuming a diet rich in protein supports muscle repair, while carbohydrates replenish glycogen stores and fats aid in hormone production.

Consistency is key to seeing progress in strength training. Regular workouts, ideally three to four times a week, ensure that the muscles are consistently challenged. Setting specific, measurable goals can help maintain motivation and track progress. For example, aiming to increase the weight lifted in a particular exercise by a certain amount over a set period provides a clear target and a sense of achievement when reached.

Listening to your body is crucial in strength training. While it is important to push your limits, it is equally important to recognize the signs of overtraining and injury. Soreness is expected, especially when starting a new routine, but persistent pain, particularly in the joints, should not be ignored. Incorporating rest days and varying the intensity and type of workouts can help prevent burnout and overuse injuries.

Strength training also offers numerous health benefits beyond muscle growth. It can improve bone density, reducing the risk of osteoporosis. It enhances metabolic rate, aiding in weight management by increasing the number of calories burned at rest. Strength training also improves insulin sensitivity, which can help manage blood sugar levels and reduce the risk of type 2 diabetes. Additionally, it can enhance cardiovascular health by lowering blood pressure and improving cholesterol levels.

Mental health benefits are another significant advantage of strength training. Exercise, including strength training, has been shown to reduce symptoms of depression and anxiety. The sense of accomplishment from lifting heavier weights or completing more repetitions can boost self-esteem and confidence. The discipline and focus required in strength training can also translate to improved concentration and mental clarity in other areas of life.

For beginners, it is advisable to start with lighter weights and focus on mastering the form before progressing to heavier loads. Working with a personal trainer or knowledgeable training partner can provide valuable guidance and feedback. Many beginners benefit from following a structured program that gradually increases the intensity and complexity of the workouts. Programs such as Starting Strength or StrongLifts 5x5 are popular for their simplicity and effectiveness in building a solid foundation.

Tracking progress is an important aspect of strength training. Keeping a workout journal or using a fitness app to log exercises, weights, and repetitions can help monitor improvements and identify areas for adjustment. Regularly reassessing goals and celebrating milestones, no matter how small, can keep motivation high and provide a sense of direction.

Strength training is a lifelong journey. As you progress, your goals and the methods to achieve them may evolve. What remains constant is the need for dedication, patience, and a willingness to learn. The principles of progressive overload, proper form, and balanced routines will guide you towards continual improvement and long-term success in your strength training endeavors.

In summary, the basics of strength training revolve around progressive overload, proper form, and a balanced mix of compound and isolation exercises. Warm-ups and recovery are crucial to prevent injury and ensure muscle growth. Consistency, goal setting, and listening to your body are key components of a successful strength training routine. Beyond muscle growth, strength training offers extensive health benefits, including improved bone density, metabolic rate, and mental health. For beginners, starting with lighter weights, focusing on form, and tracking progress will lay a strong foundation for future gains. Strength training is not just a workout regimen but a commitment to lifelong health and fitness.

Compound Movements for Maximum Efficiency

Compound movements are the cornerstone of any efficient and effective workout routine. These exercises engage multiple muscle groups and joints simultaneously, making them incredibly efficient for building strength, improving coordination, and enhancing overall fitness. Whether you're a beginner or an experienced athlete, incorporating compound movements into your routine can significantly elevate your training results.

One of the primary benefits of compound movements is their ability to maximize muscle engagement. Unlike isolation exercises, which target a single muscle group, compound movements recruit several muscles at once. Take the squat, for instance. This exercise primarily targets the quadriceps, hamstrings, and glutes, but it also engages the core, lower back, and even the muscles in the upper body to maintain stability.

This multifaceted muscle activation not only builds strength but also improves functional fitness, making everyday activities easier and more efficient.

The deadlift is another prime example of a compound movement that offers substantial benefits. It engages nearly every muscle in the body, with a particular focus on the posterior chain, including the hamstrings, glutes, and lower back. Proper form is crucial to prevent injury and maximize effectiveness. When performing a deadlift, start with your feet shoulder-width apart, grip the barbell with hands just outside your knees, and keep your back straight as you lift. The movement should be smooth and controlled, with a focus on engaging the core and keeping the bar close to your body.

In addition to muscle engagement, compound movements are highly effective for calorie burning and metabolic conditioning. Because they involve large muscle groups and multiple joints, they require more energy to perform, leading to a higher caloric expenditure both during and after the workout. This is particularly beneficial for those looking to lose weight or improve cardiovascular health. Movements like the clean and press, which combines a deadlift, row, squat, and overhead press, can elevate the heart rate and provide a full-body workout in a short amount of time.

The bench press is one of the most well-known compound movements, targeting the chest, shoulders, and triceps. To perform a bench press, lie flat on a bench with feet firmly planted on the ground. Grip the barbell slightly wider than shoulder-width apart, lower it to your chest, and then press it back up until your arms are fully extended. This exercise not only builds upper body strength but also enhances pushing power, which is essential for various sports and daily activities.

Pull-ups and chin-ups are exceptional compound movements for upper body development. These exercises primarily work the back, biceps, and shoulders while also engaging the core for stabilization. To perform a pull-up, grip the bar with palms facing away from you, hang with arms fully extended, and then pull your body up until your chin is above the bar. For chin-ups, use an underhand grip with palms facing towards you. Both variations are challenging but incredibly effective for building upper body strength and improving grip.

Lunges are another versatile compound movement that targets the legs and glutes while also engaging the core and improving balance. To perform a lunge, step forward with one leg, lower your hips until both knees are bent at a 90-degree angle, and then push back up to the starting position. Alternating legs not only ensures balanced muscle development but also adds a cardiovascular element to the exercise, especially when performed at a brisk pace.

The overhead press is a powerful compound movement for building shoulder and upper body strength. It involves lifting a barbell or dumbbells from shoulder height to overhead, engaging the shoulders, triceps, and upper chest. Proper form is essential to avoid shoulder strain. Stand with feet shoulder-width apart, grip the barbell just outside shoulder width, and press it overhead while keeping the core engaged and back straight. This movement not only builds strength but also improves shoulder stability and mobility.

Rowing exercises, such as the bent-over row or seated row, are excellent for targeting the back, biceps, and shoulders. These movements mimic the pulling motion and are crucial for developing a strong, stable upper body. To perform a bent-over row, hold a barbell or dumbbells with palms facing down, bend at the hips until your torso is nearly parallel to the floor, and then pull the weight towards your lower ribcage, squeezing the shoulder blades together. This exercise not only builds muscle but also improves posture and reduces the risk of back injuries.

The benefits of compound movements extend beyond muscle building and calorie burning. They also enhance functional fitness, which is the ability to perform everyday activities with ease and efficiency. Movements like squats, deadlifts, and lunges mimic common actions such as lifting, bending, and climbing, thereby improving overall mobility and reducing the risk of injury in daily life. Furthermore, the coordination and balance required for compound movements translate into better athletic performance and reduced injury risk in sports and recreational activities.

Incorporating compound movements into your workout routine can be done in various ways. Full-body workouts that include exercises like squats, deadlifts, bench presses, and pull-ups ensure that all major muscle groups are engaged in a single session. Alternatively, you can structure your workouts around specific muscle groups on different days, such as focusing on the lower body with squats and lunges one day and the upper body with bench presses and rows the next. This split routine allows for targeted muscle development while providing adequate recovery time between sessions.

To maximize the benefits of compound movements, it's important to follow a few key guidelines. First, always prioritize proper form over lifting heavier weights. Using correct technique not only prevents injury but also ensures that the target muscles are effectively engaged. Second, incorporate a variety of compound movements to ensure balanced muscle development and prevent overuse injuries. Finally, listen to your body and adjust your workouts as needed. Progressive overload is important, but so is allowing adequate recovery time to prevent burnout and overtraining.

One of the most compelling aspects of compound movements is their adaptability. Whether you have access to a fully equipped gym or are working out at home with minimal equipment, there are compound exercises that can fit your circumstances. Bodyweight exercises like push-ups, pull-ups, and lunges require no equipment and can be performed anywhere. Resistance bands and dumbbells offer additional versatility, allowing you to perform movements like rows, presses, and squats with varying levels of resistance.

In conclusion, compound movements are a highly efficient and effective way to build strength, burn calories, and improve overall fitness. By engaging multiple muscle groups and joints, these exercises provide a comprehensive workout that enhances functional fitness and athletic performance. Incorporating a variety of compound movements into your routine, maintaining proper form, and progressively challenging your muscles will ensure continued progress and long-term success. Whether you're lifting heavy weights or using bodyweight exercises, the principles of compound movements remain the same: engage multiple muscles, move with purpose, and strive for balance and efficiency in your training.

Bodyweight Exercises

Bodyweight exercises are a highly effective and versatile approach to fitness that can be performed anywhere, without the need for extensive equipment. They offer an excellent way to build strength, improve flexibility, and enhance cardiovascular health, making them ideal for beginners and seasoned athletes alike. The simplicity and accessibility of bodyweight exercises make them a perfect choice for those looking to start their fitness journey or seeking a convenient way to stay in shape.

One of the most fundamental bodyweight exercises is the push-up. This classic move engages the chest, shoulders, triceps, and core, providing a comprehensive upper-body workout. To perform a push-up, start in a plank position with your hands placed slightly wider than shoulder-width apart. Lower your body until your chest nearly touches the ground, then push back up to the starting position. Maintaining a straight line from head to heels is crucial for proper form and to avoid unnecessary strain on the lower back.

Squats are another cornerstone of bodyweight training, targeting the quadriceps, hamstrings, glutes, and core. Begin by standing with your feet shoulder-width apart and your toes slightly turned out. Lower your body by bending your knees and hips, keeping your chest up and your back straight. Aim to lower until your thighs are parallel to the ground, then push through your heels to return to the starting position. Squats not only build leg strength but also improve overall mobility and stability.

Lunges are excellent for developing leg strength, balance, and coordination. Start by standing tall with your feet together. Step forward with one leg and lower your body until both knees are bent at 90-degree angles, making sure your front knee does not extend past your toes. Push back up to the starting position and repeat on the other side. Alternating lunges can be performed in place or as walking lunges for added intensity. This exercise is particularly beneficial for targeting the glutes and improving unilateral strength.

The plank is a superb exercise for building core strength and stability. Begin in a push-up position but with your weight resting on your forearms instead of your hands. Keep your body in a straight line from head to heels, engaging your core and glutes to maintain this position. Hold the plank for as long as possible, aiming to increase your time gradually as your strength improves. Variations such as side planks can further challenge your core muscles and enhance oblique strength.

Burpees are a full-body exercise that combines strength and cardiovascular training. Start in a standing position, then drop into a squat and place your hands on the ground. Jump your feet back into a plank position, perform a push-up, then jump your feet back to your hands and explosively jump into the air, reaching your arms overhead. Burpees are highly effective for building endurance, strength, and explosive power, making them a staple in high-intensity interval training (HIIT) workouts.

Pull-ups and chin-ups are among the most challenging bodyweight exercises, primarily targeting the back, biceps, and shoulders. To perform a pull-up, grip a bar with your palms facing away from you and your hands slightly wider than shoulder-width apart. Hang with your arms fully extended, then pull your body up until your chin is above the bar. For chin-ups, use an underhand grip with your palms facing toward you. Both variations require significant upper-body strength and can be modified with resistance bands for assistance if necessary.

Dips are another effective upper-body exercise that targets the triceps, chest, and shoulders. Using parallel bars or a sturdy bench, position your hands shoulder-width apart and lower your body until your elbows are bent at 90 degrees. Push back up to the starting position, keeping your core engaged and your body upright. Dips can be performed with bent knees to reduce the load or with legs extended for a greater challenge.

Mountain climbers are a dynamic exercise that combines core strength with cardiovascular endurance. Start in a plank position with your hands directly under your shoulders. Drive one knee toward your chest, then quickly switch legs, mimicking a running motion while keeping your body in a plank position. This exercise not only builds core strength but also elevates the heart rate, making it an excellent addition to any cardio routine.

The bicycle crunch is an effective core exercise that targets the abdominals and obliques. Lie on your back with your hands behind your head and your legs lifted to a 90-degree angle. Bring one knee toward your chest while simultaneously twisting your torso to touch the opposite elbow to the knee. Alternate sides in a pedaling motion, ensuring that your shoulder blades lift off the ground with each twist. This movement enhances core strength and improves rotational stability.

Bodyweight exercises can be easily modified to increase or decrease difficulty, making them suitable for all fitness levels. For example, push-ups can be performed on the knees for beginners or with feet elevated for advanced practitioners. Similarly, squats can be made more challenging by adding a jump at the end of each rep or by performing single-leg variations like pistol squats.

Incorporating bodyweight exercises into your routine can be done through various training formats. Circuit training, where you perform a series of exercises back-to-back with minimal rest, is an effective way to build strength and endurance simultaneously. HIIT workouts, which involve short bursts of intense activity followed by brief rest periods, are another excellent method for maximizing the benefits of bodyweight exercises in a short amount of time.

Consistency is key when it comes to bodyweight training. Establishing a regular workout schedule and progressively challenging yourself with more reps, longer holds, or advanced variations will ensure continuous improvement. Additionally, focusing on proper form and technique is crucial to prevent injury and maximize the effectiveness of each exercise.

One of the greatest advantages of bodyweight exercises is their ability to be performed anywhere, at any time. Whether you're at home, in a park, or traveling, you can maintain your fitness routine without the need for a gym or specialized equipment. This convenience makes it easier to stay committed to your fitness goals, regardless of your circumstances.

In summary, bodyweight exercises offer a versatile and effective approach to fitness that can help you build strength, improve flexibility, and enhance cardiovascular health. By incorporating a variety of exercises and training formats, you can create a well-rounded workout routine that meets your individual needs and goals. Remember to prioritize proper form, progressively challenge yourself, and stay consistent in your efforts. With dedication and perseverance, bodyweight exercises can help you achieve and maintain a high level of fitness, no matter where you are.

Resistance Band and Dumbbell Workouts

Resistance band and dumbbell workouts provide a highly effective and versatile approach to strength training. Whether you're a beginner or a seasoned fitness enthusiast, incorporating these tools into your routine can enhance muscle growth, improve endurance, and add variety to your workouts. Their portability and ease of use make them ideal for both home and gym settings, enabling you to maintain a consistent exercise regimen wherever you are.

Resistance bands come in various levels of tension, allowing you to adjust the intensity of your workouts. They are particularly useful for targeting smaller muscle groups and enhancing flexibility. For instance, a common exercise using resistance bands is the band pull-apart. To perform this exercise, hold the band with both hands at shoulder width, keeping your arms straight in front of you. Pull the band apart by moving your hands out to the sides, squeezing your shoulder blades together, and then return to the starting position. This exercise is excellent for strengthening the upper back and shoulders.

Another effective resistance band exercise is the banded squat. Place the band around your thighs just above your knees. Stand with your feet shoulder-width apart and perform a squat by lowering your hips back and down. The resistance band adds extra tension, engaging your glutes and outer thighs more intensively. This modification not only builds leg strength but also improves overall lower body stability.

For upper body strength, the resistance band chest press can be highly effective. Anchor the band to a sturdy object behind you at chest height. Hold the ends of the band in each hand, step forward to create tension, and press your hands forward until your arms are fully extended. This movement mimics the motion of a bench press, targeting the chest, shoulders, and triceps. Adjusting the anchor point higher or lower can alter the angle of resistance, providing a comprehensive chest workout.

Dumbbells, on the other hand, offer a different set of advantages. They allow for a greater range of motion and the ability to add significant weight to exercises as you progress. One of the most fundamental dumbbell exercises is the dumbbell bench press. Lying on a bench with a dumbbell in each hand, press the weights upward until your arms are fully extended, then slowly lower them back to the starting position. This exercise primarily targets the chest, shoulders, and triceps, and can be varied with different grips and angles to target different areas of the chest.

The dumbbell row is another essential exercise, focusing on the back muscles. To perform a dumbbell row, place one knee and one hand on a bench for support, with the other foot on the ground. Hold a dumbbell in the free hand, and pull it toward your hip, squeezing your shoulder blade at the top of the movement. This exercise strengthens the upper and middle back, as well as the biceps and shoulders.

For a comprehensive lower body workout, dumbbell lunges are highly effective. Hold a dumbbell in each hand and step forward into a lunge, lowering your back knee toward the ground. Push back up to the starting position and repeat with the other leg. This exercise targets the quadriceps, hamstrings, glutes, and calves, and can be varied by stepping backward or to the side to engage different muscle groups.

Incorporating resistance bands and dumbbells into a single workout can create a balanced and dynamic routine. For example, you might start with a resistance band warm-up, performing band pull-aparts, banded squats, and chest presses to activate your muscles. Following this, you could move on to dumbbell exercises like the bench press, rows, and lunges to build strength. This combination ensures that you are engaging both the smaller stabilizing muscles and the larger muscle groups, promoting overall muscular balance and reducing the risk of injury.

When designing a resistance band and dumbbell workout, it's important to consider the principle of progressive overload. This principle involves gradually increasing the resistance or weight to continue challenging your muscles and promoting growth. For resistance bands, you can progress by using bands with higher tension or by doubling up the bands. With dumbbells, you can increase the weight or the number of repetitions and sets.

Additionally, incorporating compound movements—exercises that work multiple muscle groups at once—can maximize the efficiency of your workouts. For instance, the dumbbell clean and press is a powerful compound movement. Start with dumbbells at your sides, bend your knees slightly, and then explosively lift the dumbbells to your shoulders. From there, press the weights overhead. This exercise targets the legs, core, shoulders, and arms, providing a full-body workout in one movement.

Another effective compound exercise is the resistance band deadlift. Step on the band with your feet hip-width apart, holding the ends of the band in each hand. Hinge at the hips, keeping your back straight, and lower your torso until it's almost parallel to the ground. Then, stand back up by driving through your heels and squeezing your glutes at the top. This exercise targets the hamstrings, glutes, lower back, and core.

It's also beneficial to include functional movements that mimic everyday activities, enhancing your overall strength and mobility. The farmer's walk is a great example. Hold a heavy dumbbell in each hand and walk forward, maintaining an upright posture and engaging your core. This exercise builds grip strength, improves posture, and strengthens the entire body, particularly the core and legs.

Recovery and rest are crucial components of any workout regimen. Ensure you allow adequate time for your muscles to recover between workouts, especially when lifting heavy weights or using high-tension resistance bands. Incorporating stretching and foam rolling into your routine can aid in muscle recovery and maintain flexibility.

In summary, resistance band and dumbbell workouts offer a versatile and effective approach to strength training. By combining these tools, you can create a balanced and dynamic workout routine that targets all major muscle groups, enhances muscle growth, and improves functional strength. Remember to progress gradually, incorporate compound movements, and allow for adequate recovery to maximize the benefits of your training. With consistency and dedication, resistance band and

dumbbell workouts can help you achieve your fitness goals and
maintain a strong, healthy body.

The Importance of Flexibility

Flexibility is a crucial component of overall fitness, often overlooked in favor of strength and endurance training. However, enhancing flexibility can significantly improve performance, reduce the risk of injury, and promote longevity in physical activity. Flexibility refers to the ability of muscles and joints to move through their full range of motion. This capability is essential for performing everyday activities and athletic movements efficiently and safely.

Consider a dancer gracefully executing complex movements or a gymnast contorting their body into seemingly impossible positions. These feats highlight the importance of flexibility. While you might not aspire to such extremes, developing flexibility can enhance your quality of life and physical health. Imagine reaching for something on a high shelf without straining or bending down to tie your shoes with ease. These simple tasks become more manageable when your muscles and joints are flexible.

One of the primary benefits of flexibility is its role in injury prevention. Tight muscles can limit the range of motion in your joints, increasing the likelihood of strains and sprains. For example, if your hamstrings are tight, they might restrict the natural movement of your hips and lower back, leading to potential injury during activities like running or lifting.

Stretching exercises that target these muscles can alleviate tightness, improving mobility and reducing the risk of injury.

Flexibility also enhances athletic performance. For athletes, a greater range of motion can improve technique and efficiency in their respective sports. A golfer with flexible shoulders and hips can achieve a more powerful and accurate swing. A swimmer with flexible ankles and shoulders can glide through the water with less resistance. Even everyday fitness enthusiasts can benefit from improved flexibility. For instance, a flexible runner can take longer strides with less effort, while a weightlifter can achieve better form, reducing the risk of injury and maximizing strength gains.

Moreover, flexibility contributes to better posture and alignment. In today's world, many people spend long hours sitting at desks or looking at screens, leading to poor posture and muscle imbalances. Tight chest muscles and weak upper back muscles often cause a hunched posture, which can lead to discomfort and chronic pain. Stretching the chest muscles and strengthening the back can help counteract these effects, promoting better posture and reducing the risk of related issues.

To improve flexibility, incorporating regular stretching exercises into your fitness routine is essential. There are several types of stretching, each with its benefits. Static stretching involves holding a stretch for an extended period, typically 15-60 seconds. This type of stretching is effective for lengthening muscles and increasing range of motion. An example of static stretching is the seated hamstring stretch. Sit on the floor with your legs extended in front of you, reach for your toes, and hold the position. This stretch targets the hamstrings and lower back.

Dynamic stretching, on the other hand, involves moving parts of your body through a full range of motion. These stretches are typically performed before physical activity to prepare the muscles and joints for exercise. An example of dynamic stretching is leg swings. Stand on one leg and swing the other leg forward and backward, gradually increasing the range of motion. This movement warms up the hip flexors and hamstrings, preparing them for more intense activity.

Proprioceptive Neuromuscular Facilitation (PNF) stretching is another effective method. It involves alternating between contracting and relaxing muscles while stretching. PNF stretching usually requires a partner. For instance, to stretch the hamstrings, lie on your back with one leg extended toward the ceiling. Your partner pushes the leg toward you while you resist the movement, then relax and allow the partner to stretch the muscle further. This technique can lead to significant flexibility improvements over time.

In addition to stretching, incorporating activities like yoga and Pilates can enhance flexibility. Yoga, with its emphasis on flowing movements and holding poses, can improve flexibility, balance, and strength simultaneously. Poses like the downward dog stretch the hamstrings, calves, and shoulders, while the cobra pose stretches the chest, shoulders, and abdomen. Pilates focuses on core strength and stability, but many exercises involve stretching and lengthening muscles, promoting flexibility. The spine stretch, for example, targets the lower back and hamstrings, improving spinal mobility.

Maintaining consistent flexibility training is crucial. Flexibility gains can be lost if not regularly practiced. Aim to incorporate stretching into your routine at least three to four times a week.

Consistency is key to seeing long-term benefits. Additionally, listening to your body and avoiding overstretching is essential. Stretching should create a mild tension, not pain. Pushing too hard can lead to injury, defeating the purpose of flexibility training.

Hydration and nutrition also play roles in flexibility. Muscles are composed largely of water, and dehydration can cause them to become stiff and less pliable. Drinking adequate water throughout the day helps maintain muscle elasticity. Additionally, a diet rich in vitamins and minerals, particularly those that support muscle health like magnesium and potassium, can aid in muscle function and flexibility.

Another aspect to consider is the mind-body connection. Stress and tension can cause muscles to tighten, reducing flexibility. Practices like mindfulness and deep breathing can relax the body and mind, promoting better flexibility. For instance, taking slow, deep breaths while holding a stretch can help release tension and allow the muscle to lengthen further.

As you progress in your flexibility training, it's essential to track your improvements. Keeping a journal of your stretching routine and noting any changes in your range of motion can be motivating and help you stay on track. You might find that activities that were once challenging become easier, and your overall physical performance improves.

Incorporating flexibility training into your fitness regimen offers numerous benefits, from injury prevention and enhanced performance to better posture and overall well-being. By dedicating time to stretch regularly, you can enjoy a more active, pain-free lifestyle. Remember, flexibility is a gradual process, and consistency is crucial. Embrace the journey, listen to your body, and celebrate the improvements you make along the way.

Quick Stretching Routines

Quick stretching routines can be a game-changer for those looking to incorporate more flexibility into their daily lives without committing extensive time. These routines are designed to be efficient yet effective, providing the benefits of stretching without the need for a lengthy session. They are perfect for busy individuals who want to maintain their flexibility, prevent injury, and improve overall well-being.

Imagine you're at your desk, feeling the tension build in your shoulders and lower back after hours of sitting. A quick stretching routine can relieve that discomfort and restore your energy. Start with a simple neck stretch. Sit up straight, gently tilt your head to the right, bringing your ear towards your shoulder. Hold for 15-20 seconds, feeling the stretch along the left side of your neck. Repeat on the other side. This stretch helps alleviate tension that accumulates from prolonged periods of desk work.

Next, move on to shoulder rolls. Sit or stand with your back straight. Roll your shoulders forward in a circular motion, making sure to engage the full range of motion. Do this for about 20 seconds, then reverse the direction. Shoulder rolls help increase blood flow to the shoulder muscles, reducing stiffness and promoting relaxation.

For your upper back, try the seated spinal twist. Sit with your feet flat on the floor and your back straight. Place your right hand on the back of your chair and your left hand on your right knee. Gently twist your torso to the right, looking over your shoulder. Hold for 15-20 seconds, then switch sides. This stretch helps improve spinal mobility and relieve tension in the upper back.

To address lower back tightness, the seated forward bend is highly effective. While sitting, extend your legs straight in front of you. Reach forward with both hands, aiming to touch your toes or as far as you comfortably can. Hold for 15-20 seconds. This stretch targets the hamstrings and lower back, areas that often become tight from prolonged sitting.

Standing stretches can also be incorporated into quick routines. The standing quad stretch, for instance, is excellent for targeting the front of the thighs. Stand on one leg, using a chair or wall for support if needed. Grab your opposite ankle with your hand, pulling your heel towards your glutes. Hold for 15-20 seconds, then switch legs. This stretch helps maintain flexibility in the quadriceps, which is crucial for activities like walking and running.

The standing calf stretch is another valuable addition. Stand facing a wall with your hands pressed against it at shoulder height. Step one foot back, keeping it straight and pressing the heel into the ground. Bend your front knee slightly and lean forward, feeling the stretch in your back calf. Hold for 15-20 seconds, then switch legs. This stretch helps prevent tightness in the calves, which can lead to issues like plantar fasciitis.

Incorporating dynamic stretches into your quick routines can further enhance flexibility and prepare your muscles for more vigorous activity. Leg swings are a great example. Stand on one leg, using a wall or chair for balance. Swing your other leg forward and backward, gradually increasing the range of motion. Perform this for 20-30 seconds, then switch legs. Leg swings help warm up the hip flexors and hamstrings, making them ideal before a workout.

Arm circles can also be included in dynamic stretching. Stand with your feet shoulder-width apart and extend your arms out to the sides at shoulder height. Make small circles with your arms, gradually increasing the size. Perform this for 20-30 seconds, then reverse the direction. Arm circles help improve shoulder mobility and increase blood flow to the upper body.

To incorporate a full-body stretch, try the standing side stretch. Stand with your feet together and raise your arms overhead, clasping your hands together. Lean to the right, feeling the stretch along the left side of your body. Hold for 15-20 seconds, then switch sides. This stretch targets the obliques, lats, and hip muscles, promoting overall flexibility and balance.

For those with a bit more time, integrating quick yoga poses can be highly beneficial. The cat-cow stretch, for example, is excellent for spinal flexibility. Start on your hands and knees in a tabletop position. Inhale, arching your back and lifting your head and tailbone towards the ceiling (cow pose). Exhale, rounding your spine and tucking your chin to your chest (cat pose). Repeat this flow for 30-60 seconds. The cat-cow stretch helps warm up the spine and improve overall back flexibility.

The downward dog is another effective yoga pose. Start on your hands and knees, then lift your hips towards the ceiling, forming an inverted V shape with your body. Keep your hands shoulder-width apart and your feet hip-width apart. Hold for 20-30 seconds, feeling the stretch in your hamstrings, calves, and shoulders. The downward dog is a great full-body stretch that can be incorporated into any quick routine.

For a hip opener, the butterfly stretch is simple yet effective. Sit with your feet together and your knees bent out to the sides. Hold your feet with your hands and gently press your knees towards the floor. Hold for 15-20 seconds. This stretch targets the inner thighs and hips, which can become tight from prolonged sitting or physical activity.

Incorporating these stretches into a daily routine doesn't require much time, but the benefits are substantial. These quick routines can be done in the morning to wake up the body, during breaks at work to alleviate tension, or in the evening to wind down. Consistency is key, and even a few minutes each day can lead to significant improvements in flexibility and overall well-being.

For those new to stretching, it's important to start slowly and listen to your body. Stretching should never cause pain, only a gentle pull or mild discomfort. Over time, as flexibility improves, you can gradually increase the duration and intensity of your stretches.

Incorporating quick stretching routines into your daily life can enhance flexibility, reduce the risk of injury, and improve overall physical and mental well-being. These routines are easy to perform, require no special equipment, and can be done anywhere, making them accessible for everyone. By dedicating just a few minutes each day to stretching, you can enjoy the benefits of a more flexible, resilient, and healthy body.

Dynamic Warm-Ups and Cool-Downs

Dynamic warm-ups and cool-downs are essential components of any effective fitness regimen, designed to prepare your body for exercise and aid in recovery afterward. These routines are more than just a formality; they play a crucial role in enhancing performance and preventing injuries. Whether you're embarking on a high-intensity workout or a gentle yoga session, incorporating dynamic movements at the beginning and end of your exercise can make a significant difference.

Imagine you're about to start a run. Instead of jumping straight into a sprint, you begin with a series of dynamic warm-up exercises. Start with high knees: stand tall and lift one knee to your chest, then quickly switch to the other knee, mimicking a running motion. This exercise warms up the hip flexors, quads, and core, gradually increasing your heart rate. Continue this for 30 seconds to a minute.

Next, transition to butt kicks. Stand and jog in place, bringing your heels up to touch your glutes. This movement targets the hamstrings and helps loosen up the muscles in the back of your legs. Perform butt kicks for another 30 seconds to a minute. These exercises are not only effective but also fun, injecting a sense of play into your routine.

Lateral leg swings are another excellent dynamic warm-up. Stand next to a wall or hold onto something for balance. Swing one leg side to side, gradually increasing the range of motion. This movement helps loosen up the hip joints and improve overall leg flexibility. Perform 10-15 swings on each leg.

Arm circles are a fantastic way to warm up the upper body. Extend your arms out to the sides at shoulder height and make small circles, gradually increasing the size. Switch directions after 15-20 seconds. This exercise increases blood flow to the shoulder muscles and prepares them for more strenuous activity.

Incorporating dynamic stretches like these before a workout helps increase blood flow to the muscles, elevates the heart rate, and activates the nervous system. The goal is to prepare the body for the specific movements it will perform during the workout. For instance, if you're about to lift weights, include dynamic stretches that mimic lifting movements, such as arm swings and torso twists.

Torso twists are particularly beneficial for activating the core and warming up the spine. Stand with your feet shoulder-width apart and hold your arms out in front of you, elbows bent. Twist your torso to the right, then to the left, in a controlled manner. Perform 10-15 twists on each side. This movement helps improve spinal mobility and prepares the core for more intense activity.

Another effective dynamic warm-up is the walking lunge with a twist. Step forward into a lunge position, then twist your torso towards the lead leg. Return to standing and repeat on the other side. This exercise warms up the hip flexors, quads, and core, while also improving balance and coordination. Perform 10-12 lunges on each side.

After completing your workout, it's equally important to cool down properly. A well-structured cool-down helps reduce muscle soreness, lower the heart rate gradually, and promote recovery. Begin with a gentle jog or brisk walk for 3-5 minutes to bring down your heart rate.

Follow this with dynamic stretches that focus on the muscles you just worked. For example, if you've completed a leg workout, incorporate dynamic hamstring stretches. Stand with your feet hip-width apart, bend forward at the hips, and reach towards the ground, then come back up. Repeat this movement 10-15 times. This helps lengthen the hamstrings and promotes flexibility.

Another effective cool-down exercise is the standing quad stretch. Stand on one leg and grab your opposite ankle, pulling your heel towards your glutes. Hold for a few seconds, then switch legs. Repeat this stretch 5-10 times on each leg to help alleviate tension in the quadriceps.

For the upper body, dynamic chest stretches are beneficial. Stand with your feet shoulder-width apart and extend your arms out to the sides. Slowly bring your arms together in front of you, then open them back out. Perform 10-15 repetitions. This stretch helps open up the chest muscles and promote better posture.

Cooling down with dynamic movements helps maintain the flexibility and mobility of your muscles without causing them to tighten up. It also aids in the removal of waste products like lactic acid, which can build up during exercise and contribute to muscle soreness.

In addition to these physical benefits, dynamic cool-downs provide a moment to reflect on your workout and connect with your body. Pay attention to how your muscles feel and take note of any areas that might need extra attention in future workouts.

For those engaging in high-intensity interval training (HIIT) or cardiovascular workouts, incorporating active recovery into your cool-down can be particularly beneficial. Active recovery involves performing low-intensity exercises that keep the body moving while promoting recovery. Examples include light jogging, cycling at a slow pace, or performing gentle bodyweight exercises like squats or lunges.

One effective active recovery exercise is the gentle bodyweight squat. Stand with your feet shoulder-width apart and lower your body into a squat position, then return to standing. Perform this movement slowly and with control for 10-15 repetitions. This helps keep the blood flowing to the legs and reduces muscle stiffness.

Another active recovery option is the arm and shoulder stretch. Stand with your feet hip-width apart and extend one arm across your body, using the opposite hand to gently pull it closer to your chest. Hold for a few seconds, then switch arms. Perform 5-10 stretches on each side to help release tension in the shoulders.

Incorporating yoga poses into your cool-down can also be highly beneficial. Poses like the child's pose and the cat-cow stretch help relax the muscles and promote flexibility. For the child's pose, kneel on the floor with your big toes touching and your knees apart. Sit back on your heels and extend your arms forward, lowering your forehead to the ground. Hold this pose for 30-60 seconds, breathing deeply.

The cat-cow stretch is another excellent cool-down exercise. Start on your hands and knees in a tabletop position. Inhale, arching your back and lifting your head and tailbone towards the ceiling (cow pose). Exhale, rounding your spine and tucking your chin to your chest (cat pose). Repeat this flow for 30-60 seconds to help stretch and relax the spine.

By incorporating dynamic warm-ups and cool-downs into your fitness routine, you can enhance your performance, prevent injuries, and promote overall well-being. These routines are simple to perform, require no special equipment, and can be adapted to suit any workout. Whether you're a beginner or an experienced athlete, making dynamic movements a regular part of your exercise regimen will yield significant benefits. Remember to listen to your body, start slowly, and gradually increase the intensity and duration of your stretches as your flexibility improves.